American Brain Tumor Association

2720 River Road, Suite 146
Des Plaines, IL 60018-4110
E-mail: info@abta.org

847.827.9910
800.886.2282
Fax: 847.827.9918

We are proud to make available this 25th Anniversary edition of

A PRIMER OF BRAIN TUMORS

A Patient's Reference Manual

Sharing knowledge, Sharing hope

Learning you or your loved one has a tumor in the brain or spine is frightening because, if you are like most of us, you haven't faced a serious situation like this before. You may know little about tumors, and even less about the brain. You might be confused about the new terms you are hearing, angry because you are forced to make decisions you are not prepared for, and dazed by all the changes in your life.

The American Brain Tumor Association wrote this book to help you, your family and your friends learn about, and better understand, brain tumors. We hope this knowledge will offer you a degree of comfort and help you feel more in control of your life.

How to use this booklet

This **Primer** is intended to be a reference manual. For background information, we suggest everyone read the following:

- ▸ Chapter 1: Parts of the Brain
- ▸ Chapter 2: Brain Tumor Basics
- ▸ Chapter 5: Symptoms

Then, refer to the other chapters as you need them.

This Primer is dedicated to the memory of
_____ **Jerome Braverman and Florence Braverman**

Jerome served as president of the Association from 1979 to 1981 and his efforts made the first edition of this publication possible. Active in a variety of civic and charitable causes, Jerry often went out of his way to help those in need. His broad shoulders, patient ear, and soothing voice are missed.

Florence devoted herself to responding personally with notes of thanks to the thousands of people who supported the Association's work with their contributions and good wishes. A caring and generous person, the loss of Florence's kindness and understanding leaves a void that cannot be filled.

_____ **Acknowledgments**

We are extremely grateful to the literally thousands of people whose generosity has made this Primer possible. We particularly appreciate the contribution of Gail Segal, Chicago, Illinois for writing and designing this book, and the ABTA staff who contributed their expertise.

Contents

continued

List of Illustrations

Illustration Credits

[1] *LifeART* Collection Images, Copyright © 1998 Williams & Wilkins, A Waverly Company, Baltimore.

[2] Burger, Scheithauer and Vogel. *Surgical Pathology of the Nervous System and its Coverings.* 3rd edition. Churchill Livingstone, New York, 1991. Diagram reproduced with permission.

With Gratitude to Our Generous Sponsors

Abbott Laboratories Fund

Barrow Neurological Institute at St. Joseph's Hospital & Medical Center, Phoenix

Bear Necessities Pediatric Cancer Foundation

Cedars-Sinai Neurosurgical Institute

Chicago Institute of Neurosurgery and Neuroresearch

Children's Medical Center of Dallas

Cleveland Clinic

Colgate-Palmolive Company

Department of Neurosurgery at NYU Medical Center

Section of Neurosurgery at the Milton S. Hershey Medical Center, Penn State Geisinger Health System, Pennsylvania

The Hassenfeld Foundation

Henry Ford Midwest Neuro-Oncology Center, Henry Ford Health System, Detroit

The Kapoor Charitable Foundation

Lands' End

Maryland Brain Tumor Center at University of Maryland Medical Center

Mayo Cancer Center

Memorial Sloan-Kettering Cancer Center

Midwest Children's Brain Tumor Center of Lutheran General Hospital, Illinois

Morgan Stanley Dean Witter

The Nalco Foundation

The Cancer Center at New England Medical Center – A Lifespan Partner

Newman's Own

Judy F. Oliphant, Remembering Hugh

Platinum Technology

University of Arkansas Medical Center

Jerry E. Windham

With Gratitude to Our Technical Reviewers

Mitchel S. Berger, MD
Neurosurgery
University of California
San Francisco, California

Steven Brem, MD
Neurosurgery
H. Lee Moffitt Cancer Center
Tampa, Florida

Jan C. Buckner, MD
Medical Oncology
Mayo Clinic
Rochester, Minnesota

Peter C. Burger, MD
Neuro-Pathology
The Johns Hopkins Medical Institutions
Baltimore, Maryland

Central Brain Tumor Registry of the United States
Chicago, Illinois

The Childhood Brain Tumor Foundation
Germantown, Maryland

Richard S. Kaplan, MD
Clinical Investigations Branch
National Cancer Institute
Bethesda, Maryland

Teresa E. Omert, RN, MS, CNRN
Neuroscience Clinical Nurse Specialist
Chicago Institute of Neurosurgery & Neuroresearch
Chicago, Illinois

Roger J. Packer, MD
Pediatric Neurology
Children's National Medical Center
Washington, DC

Nina A. Paleologos, MD
Neuro-Oncology
Evanston Hospital
Evanston, Illinois

Roberta Stine-Reyes, RN, MS, CNRN
Clinical Nurse Specialist Neurosurgery
University of Chicago Medical Center
Chicago, Illinois

W. K. Alfred Yung, MD
Neuro-Oncology
UT MD Anderson Cancer Center
Houston, Texas

American Brain Tumor Association ▲ 800/886-2282

Chapter 1

Parts of the Brain

Living creatures are made up of cells. Groups of cells, similar in appearance and with the same function, form tissue. The *brain* is a soft, spongy mass of nerve and supportive tissue connected to the *spinal cord*. Nerves in the brain and spinal cord transmit messages throughout the body. The brain and spinal cord together form the *central nervous system (CNS)*.

The central nervous system is the core of our existence. It controls our *personality*—thoughts, memory, intelligence, speech and understanding, emotions; *senses*—vision, hearing, taste, smell, touch; *basic body functions*—breathing, heart beat, blood pressure; how we *function in our environment*—movement, balance, coordination.

A knowledge of the parts of the brain and spine will help you understand the symptoms of brain tumors, how they are diagnosed, and how they are treated.

▲ Basal Ganglia

These are masses of nerve cells deep within the brain at the base of the cerebral hemispheres.

▲ Brain Stem

It is the bottom-most portion of the brain, connecting the cerebrum with the spinal cord. The *midbrain, pons, medulla oblongata* and *reticular formation* are all part of the brain stem.

▲ Cerebellopontine Angle

The angle between the pons and the cerebellum.

▲ Cerebellum

The cerebellum is the second largest area of the brain. It consists of two hemispheres or halves. The cerebellum is connected to the brain stem.

▲ Cerebrospinal Fluid (CSF)

CSF is the clear, watery fluid made in the ventricles that bathes and cushions the brain and spinal cord. It circulates through the ventricles and the subarachnoid space.

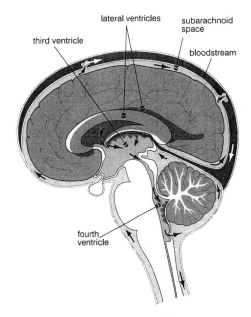

Cerebrospinal Fluid Flow

▲ Cerebrum/Cerebral Hemispheres

The largest area of the brain is the cerebrum which consists of the right and left hemispheres. In general, the right cerebral hemisphere controls the left side of the body and the left cerebral hemisphere controls the right side of the body.

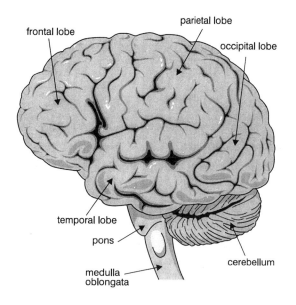

frontal lobe
parietal lobe
occipital lobe
temporal lobe
pons
medulla oblongata
cerebellum

Major Parts of the Brain

Each hemisphere is comprised of four sections called *lobes*: frontal, parietal, temporal, and occipital. Each lobe controls a specific group of activities.

The outer layer of the cerebrum is made up of *gray matter*— the bodies of nerve cells. Nerve cells control brain activity.

The inner portion of the cerebrum is mostly *white matter*—nerve fibers called axons. White matter carries information between nerve cells by conducting electrical impulses.

▲ Choroid Plexus

The choroid plexus produces spinal fluid, which flows through the *ventricles* and *meninges* surrounding the brain and spinal cord.

▲ Corpus Callosum

The corpus callosum is made of nerve fibers, deep in the brain, that pass through and connect the two halves of the cerebral hemispheres.

▲ Cranial Nerves

There are 12 pair of cranial nerves. Their functions are described in the illustration at the bottom of this page.

▲ Glial Tissue (Neuroglia)

Glia is the supportive tissue of the brain. The most common glial cells are *astrocytes* and *oligodendrocytes*. Unlike nerves, glia can reproduce itself.

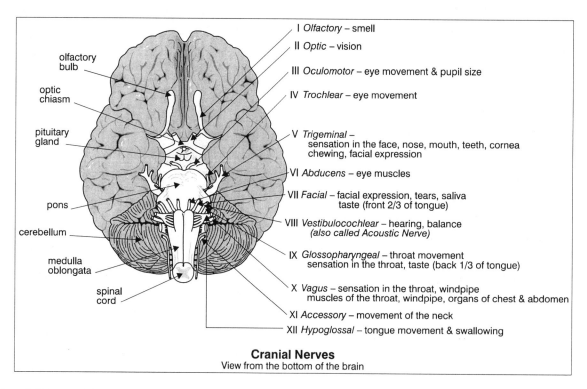

olfactory bulb
optic chiasm
pituitary gland
pons
cerebellum
medulla oblongata
spinal cord

I *Olfactory* – smell

II *Optic* – vision

III *Oculomotor* – eye movement & pupil size

IV *Trochlear* – eye movement

V *Trigeminal* – sensation in the face, nose, mouth, teeth, cornea chewing, facial expression

VI *Abducens* – eye muscles

VII *Facial* – facial expression, tears, saliva taste (front 2/3 of tongue)

VIII *Vestibulocochlear* – hearing, balance (also called Acoustic Nerve)

IX *Glossopharyngeal* – throat movement sensation in the throat, taste (back 1/3 of tongue)

X *Vagus* – sensation in the throat, windpipe muscles of the throat, windpipe, organs of chest & abdomen

XI *Accessory* – movement of the neck

XII *Hypoglossal* – tongue movement & swallowing

Cranial Nerves
View from the bottom of the brain

Glia is the origin of the largest percentage of brain tumors.

Astrocytes are involved with the blood brain barrier and brain metabolism. Oligodendrocytes maintain the myelin covering of nerve cells. Myelin helps transmit information between nerve cells.

▲ Hypothalamus

The hypothalamus makes up part of the wall of the third ventricle and is the base of the optic chiasm.

▲ Limbic System

The limbic system, together with the hypo-

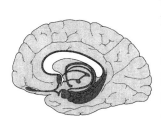

thalamus, controls hunger, thirst, emotional reactions, and biological rhythms. It is also involved with the endocrine and autonomic motor systems.

▲ Medulla Oblongata

The medulla oblongata, a part of the brain stem, connects the brain with the spinal cord. It contains the origins of the 9th, 10th, 11th, and 12th cranial nerves.

▲ Meninges

The meninges are three, thin membranes that completely cover the brain and the spinal cord. Spinal fluid flows in the space between two of the membranes.

▲ Midbrain

The midbrain is the short portion of the brain stem between the pons and the cerebral hemispheres. The top of the midbrain is called the *tectum* (or tectal area). The 3rd and 4th cranial nerves originate in the midbrain.

▲ Optic Chiasm

The optic chiasm is the area under the hypothalamus where each of the two optic nerves crosses over to the opposite side, forming an X shape.

▲ Pineal Gland

The pineal gland lies below the corpus callosum. It produces the hormone melatonin. This hormone is believed to control the biological rhythms of the body.

▲ Pituitary Gland

The pituitary gland is attached to, and receives messages from, the *hypothalamus*. The pituitary

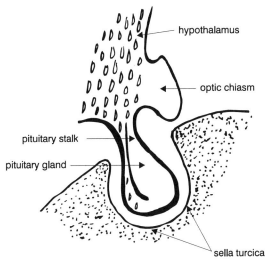

The Pituitary Gland

gland is composed of two lobes, the anterior and the posterior. Several hormones are produced by the pituitary including prolactin, corticotropin, and growth hormone.

▲ Pons

The pons, a part of the brain stem, contains the origins of the 5th, 6th, 7th, and 8th cranial nerves.

▲ Posterior Fossa (infratentorium)

This is the area within the skull that contains the *cerebellum* and the *brain stem*. The tentorium separates the posterior fossa from the cerebral hemispheres.

▲ Reticular Formation

The reticular formation is the central core of the brain stem. It connects with all parts of the brain and brain stem.

▲ Sellar Region (also Suprasellar, Parasellar)

The sellar region is the area around the sella turcica. The sella turcica is the hollow of skull bone that contains the pituitary gland.

▲ Skull Base

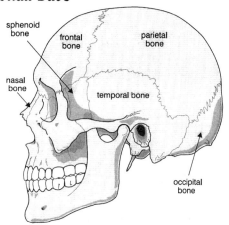

The Skull

Skull base refers to the bony areas that support the bottom of the frontal lobes, the bottom of the temporal lobes, and the brain stem and cerebellum.

▲ Spinal Cord

The spinal cord is made up of nerve fibers. It begins in the medulla oblongata of the brain and continues through the hollow center of the vertebrae (the bones of the spine). The spinal cord is covered by the meninges. Cerebrospinal fluid flows through the meninges.

▲ Supratentorium

The supratentorium is the area above the tentorium containing the cerebral hemispheres.

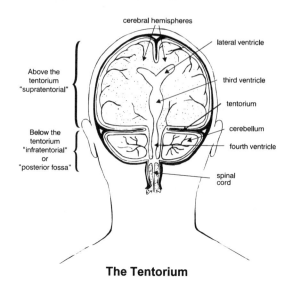

The Tentorium

▲ Tentorium

The tentorium is a flap of meninges separating the cerebral hemispheres from the structures in the posterior fossa.

▲ Thalamus

The thalamus surrounds the third *ventricle*.

▲ Ventricles

Four connected cavities called ventricles contain

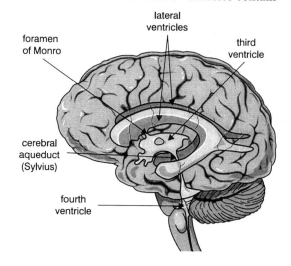

The Ventricles

choroid plexus which produce spinal fluid. The fluid flows through the ventricles and the subarachnoid space of the meninges.

There are two lateral ventricles, one in each cerebral hemisphere. The third ventricle is beneath the corpus callosum and surrounded by the thalamus. The fourth ventricle is an expansion of the central canal of the medulla oblongata.

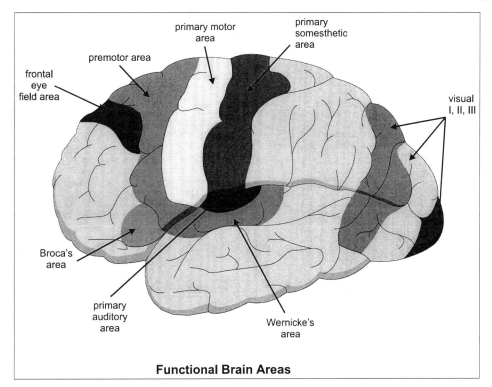

Functional Brain Areas

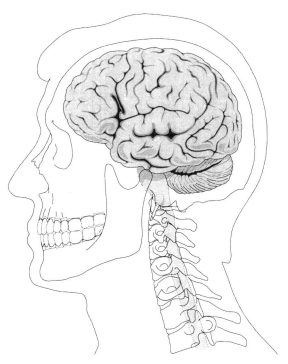

View of the Brain within the Skull

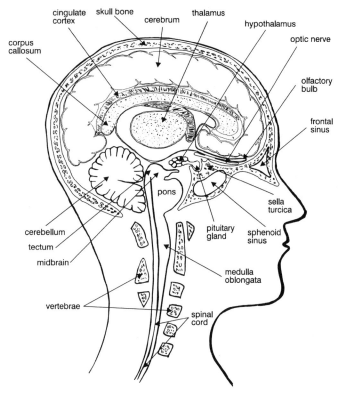

Cross Section of the Brain

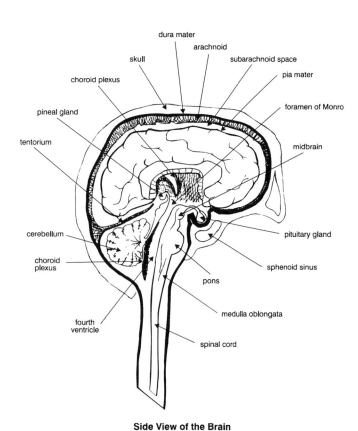

Side View of the Brain

Central Nervous System

Chapter 2

Brain Tumor Basics

The adult body normally forms new cells only when they are needed to replace old or damaged ones. Infants and children form new cells to complete their development in addition to those needed for repair. A tumor develops if normal or abnormal cells multiply when they are not needed.

A brain tumor is a mass of unnecessary, and often abnormal, cells growing in the brain.

Benign vs Malignant

When doctors describe brain tumors, they often use the words benign or malignant. Those descriptions refer to the degree of malignancy or aggressiveness of a brain tumor. It is not always easy to classify a brain tumor as "benign" or "malignant." And many factors other than the pathological analysis contribute to the outcome.

▲ Benign brain tumors

A benign brain tumor consists of very slow growing cells, has distinct borders, and rarely spreads. When viewed microscopically, the cells have an almost normal appearance. Surgery alone might be an effective treatment for this type of tumor. A brain tumor composed of benign cells, but located in a vital area, can be considered to be life-threatening—even though the tumor and its cells wouldn't be classified as malignant.

▲ Malignant brain tumors

A malignant brain tumor is life-threatening, invasive and often grows rapidly. Other malignant tumors are invasive but grow more slowly. Malignant brain tumors are often called **brain cancer**. Since primary brain tumors rarely spread outside the brain and spinal cord, they do not exactly fit the general definition of cancer.

Cancer is a disease defined by the following characteristics:

- ▸ unregulated growth of abnormal cells
- ▸ invasion of local structures thus interfering with normal functioning
- ▸ spread to distant locations in the body

Brain tumors can be malignant if they:

- ▸ have the characteristics of cancer cells or
- ▸ are located in a critical part of the brain or
- ▸ are causing life-threatening damage

Malignant brain tumors that are cancerous can spread to other locations in the brain and spine. They rarely spread to other parts of the body. They invade and destroy healthy tissue. They lack distinct borders due to their tendency to send "roots" into nearby normal tissue. They can also shed cells that travel to distant parts of the brain and spine by way of the cerebrospinal fluid. Some malignant tumors, however, do remain localized.

Primary Brain Tumors

A tumor that starts in the brain is a primary brain tumor. *Glioblastoma multiforme, astrocytoma* and *medulloblastoma* are examples of primary brain tumors.

Metastatic Brain Tumors

Cancer cells that begin growing elsewhere in the body and then travel to the brain form metastatic

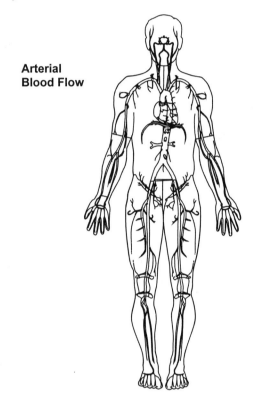

Arterial Blood Flow

brain tumors. For example, cancers of the lung, breast, colon and skin (melanoma) frequently spread to the brain. All metastatic brain tumors are, by definition, malignant.

Tumor Names

Tumors are diagnosed and then named based on a classification system. Brain tumor classification is explained in Appendix A (page 114), and information about most tumor types is contained in Chapter 7, *Types of Brain and Spinal Cord Tumors* (page 36).

Your **diagnosis and the name of your tumor might be changed**. There are several factors that might cause the change in diagnosis:

- Inspecting only a small sample of the tumor, such as that obtained by a needle biopsy,

might not be representative of the whole tumor.

- Tumors do not always remain static. They can undergo transformation, usually to a higher grade. If that occurs, the name of the tumor might change. A *grade III anaplastic/ malignant astrocytoma* could become a *glioblastoma* or *grade IV astrocytoma*.
- You should also be aware that classification of brain tumors by the pathologist is a subjective procedure that isn't always straightforward. Different pathologists might disagree about the classification and grade of the same tumor.

Tumor Grading

There are three reasons for grading tumors—to facilitate communication, to plan treatment and to predict outcome. The grade of a tumor indicates its degree of malignancy. Grade is assigned based on the tumor's microscopic appearance using some or all of the following criteria:

- similarity to normal cells (*atypia*)
- rate of growth (*mitotic index*)
- indications of uncontrolled growth—dead tumor cells in the center of the tumor (*necrosis*)
- potential for invasion and/or spread (*infiltration*) based on whether or not it has a definitive margin (*diffuse or focal*)
- blood supply (*vascularity*)

Using the **WHO** (World Health Organization) grading system, grade I tumors are the least malignant and are usually associated with long-term survival. The tumors grow slowly, and have an almost normal appearance when viewed through a microscope. Surgery alone might be an effective treatment for this grade of tumor. *Pilocytic astrocytoma, craniopharyngioma,* and many tumors of neurons, for example, *gangliocytoma* and *ganglioglioma*, are examples of grade I tumors.

Grade II tumors are relatively slow growing but have a slightly abnormal microscopic appearance. They can invade adjacent normal tissue and recur. Sometimes these tumors recur as a higher grade.

Grade III tumors are, by definition, malignant, although there isn't always a sharp distinction between a grade II and a grade III tumor. The cells of a grade III tumor are actively reproducing abnormal cells and infiltrate adjacent normal brain tissue. These tumors tend to recur, often as a higher grade.

The most malignant tumors are given a grade of IV. They reproduce rapidly, have a bizarre appearance when viewed under the microscope and infiltrate widely. These tumors induce the formation of new blood vessels so they can maintain their rapid growth. They also have areas of dead cells in their center. The *glioblastoma multiforme* is the most common example of a grade IV tumor.

Tumors often contain several grades of cells. The highest or most malignant grade of cell found when the tumor tissue is examined under a microscope determines the grade, even if most of the tumor is a lower grade.

Some tumors undergo change. A benign growth might become malignant. In some tumors, a lower-grade tumor might recur as a higher-grade tumor. Only rarely, after treatment, do higher-grade tumors become lower-grade.

———

All grading systems have inherent difficulties—they are not precise.

▸ criteria used to assign grades are subject to interpretation by each pathologist

▸ tumors are not uniform, and the sample examined might not be representative of the entire tumor

Tumor Staging (Primary Brain Tumors)

"Staging" determines if a tumor has spread beyond the site of its origin. In cancers such as breast, colon or prostate, this is primarily accomplished by a pathologist's examination of nearby tissue such as lymph nodes. In those cancers, staging is a basic part of the diagnostic work-up.

Staging for central nervous system (CNS) tumors is usually inferred from scan images or by examining the cerebrospinal fluid. Scans taken after surgery are used to determine if there is remaining tumor and the possibility of distant spread within the central nervous system. CNS tumors that are especially prone to spread are studied with both scan images and laboratory tests. For example, patients with *medulloblastoma* will have their cerebrospinal fluid examined for the presence of tumor cells. Those patients will also have scans of their spinal cord because of that tumor's tendency to spread there.

Staging information often influences treatment recommendations and prognosis.

Prognosis

Prognosis means prediction. It is an educated guess about the future course of a disease in a specific individual.

Prognosis is based on the type of tumor, its grade, location and spread (if any), the age of the patient, how long the patient had symptoms before the tumor was diagnosed, how much the tumor has affected the patient's ability to function, and the extent of surgery if surgery was performed.

The type of therapy is also instrumental. Certain tumors, although malignant, can be cured by radiation therapy. Others, by virtue of their location, may ultimately be lethal in spite of their "benign" appearance under the microscope.

Chapter 3

Facts and Statistics — 2000

Brain tumors don't discriminate. Primary brain tumors occur in people of all ages, but they are statistically more frequent in two age groups—children under the age of 20, and older adults. Metastatic brain tumors are much more common in adults.

Spinal cord tumors are less common than brain tumors. Although they affect people of all ages, they occur most frequently in young and middle-aged adults.

The facts and statistics below include **brain and spinal cord tumors** (central nervous system tumors).

Incidence in the United States

▲ ALL brain tumors

- Over 185,000 people will be diagnosed with a brain or spinal cord tumor in the year 2000.
- Of that number, about 35,000 will be primary brain tumors and 150,000 will be metastatic tumors.
- The number of primary tumors is based on an incidence rate of 12.8 per 100,000 people, [1] and a projected 2000 census of 275,306,000. The number of metastatic tumors is based on 10-15% of patients with cancer developing brain metastasis, [2] and 1,220,000 new cases of cancer per year. [3]
- Of the 35,000 people that will be diagnosed with a primary brain tumor in 2000, the gender breakdown will be:
  Males: 13.53 per 100,000
  Females: 12.25 per 100,000 [1]

▲ INCIDENCE trends

- Improvements in diagnosis explain the previously reported increase in the number of brain tumors. Incidence appears to be leveling off in nearly every age group except for those 85 years of age and older.

▲ PRIMARY brain tumors

- **By age,** the most common primary brain tumors in **adults** are:
  Ages 20-34 *pituitary tumor*
  Ages 35-44 *meningioma*
  Ages 45-74 *glioblastoma*
  Ages 75 and older *meningioma* [1]
- **By tumor type,** the most common primary brain tumors are:
  meningioma—24%
  glioblastoma—23%
  astrocytoma, pituitary tumors—8% each
  acoustic neuroma, neurilemmoma—6%
  anaplastic astrocytoma, lymphoma—4% each
  oligodendroglioma—3%

▲ METASTATIC brain tumors

- Metastatic brain tumors are most commonly formed by breast, lung and melanoma cancers.

▲ CHILDREN

- Brain and spinal cord tumors are the second most frequent malignancy of childhood.[4] (The leukemias are first.)

▸ About 2,200 children will be diagnosed with a brain tumor in 2000.[4]

▸ **By age,** the most common primary brain tumors in **children** are:
Ages 0-9 *primitive neuroectodermal tumors (PNETs) / medulloblastoma*
Ages 10-14 *astrocytomas*
Ages 15-19 *pilocytic astrocytomas* [1]

Mortality

▸ Primary malignant brain tumors cause 2% or 13,000 of the deaths due to cancer in the United States each year.[3]

▸ More men (7,100) than women (5,900) die of malignant brain tumors annually.[3]

▸ Brain tumors represent 23% of cancer-related deaths in male children under the age of 20, and 25% of cancer-related deaths in female children under the age of 20.[3]

Brain tumors are the:

▸ **2nd** most common cause of cancer death in children under the age of 20 [3]

▸ **3rd** most common cause of cancer death in people ages 20 to 39 [3]

▸ **3rd** most common cause of cancer death in males ages 20-39 [3]

▸ **4th** leading cause of cancer death in women ages 20-39 [3]

For Additional Information

Visit the Central Brain Tumor Registry of the United States (CBTRUS) at their website: www.cbtrus.org

In 1990, the American Brain Tumor Association conducted a feasibility study to determine the practicality of forming a registry to collect statistics for all brain tumors.

The results of the study highlighted the need for and feasibility of such a registry. The American Brain Tumor Association provided organizational and financial support to form the new entity.

CBTRUS was incorporated as a not-for-profit organization in 1992 to provide a resource for gathering and circulating current information on all primary brain tumors—benign and malignant—for the purposes of:

▸ describing incidence and survival patterns
▸ evaluating diagnosis and treatment
▸ facilitating etiologic (causation) studies
▸ establishing awareness of the disease
▸ and, ultimately, for the prevention of all brain tumors

State or regional tumor registries obtain information about brain tumor patients from hospitals in their area. CBTRUS began by collecting information from four registries that were already collecting data on benign and malignant brain tumors.

Using preliminary data, CBTRUS conducted studies to determine diagnostic accuracy and data completeness. They now have the voluntary collaboration of 11 state registries.

The data collected is used to define incidence rates of all primary brain tumors and can be used by researchers to support grant applications and identify geographic clusters of patients.

For more information, contact CBTRUS ▾ 3333 West 47th Street ▾ Chicago, Illinois 60632 ▾ (773) 579-0021 ▾ Fax (630) 655-1756 ▾ E-mail: cbtrus@aol.com

Legend

▸ **CBTRUS**
Central **B**rain **T**umor **R**egistry of the **US**
Uses existing data from SEER and NAACCR to describe brain tumors in the United States.
1) SEER—malignant brain tumor incidence, mortality and survival data
2) NAACCR—malignant and benign brain tumor incidence, mortality and survival data (eleven of thirty-four registries provide data to CBTRUS)

▸ **Classification**
A grouping based on shared characteristics. Brain tumors are classified by their histology on the assumption that each type of tumor results from the abnormal growth of a specific cell type. A

good classification system will help predict a tumor's behavior, the patient's prognosis and serve as a guide to treatment. Classification is the basis for communication.

▸ **Histology**

Microscopic anatomy. Characteristics of cells observed under the microscope.

▸ **Incidence**

The number of newly diagnosed people in one year.

▸ **Mortality**

The number of people who died of a brain tumor in one year.

▸ **NAACCR**

North American Association of Central Cancer Registries

The thirty-four population-based cancer registries in North America

▸ **Prevalence**

The number of people in the US currently surviving with a specific disease. The total number of brain tumor survivors is not known.

▸ **Rate**

A measure of the amount of a disease in a specific population. It is calculated by counting the number of patients with the disease and dividing by the total population at risk. Rates are expressed as a unit of person-years (usually 100,000). A person-year is one person for one year.

▸ **SEER**

Surveillance, Epidemiology and End Results
SEER is the source of most of the published cancer statistics in the US. It is a program of the National Cancer Institute, formed under the National Cancer Act of 1971. It collects and analyzes information on cancer incidence, mortality and survival in the US. (Benign brain tumors are not included in SEER data.)

Data are collected from cancer registries representing about 14% of the total US population. (Connecticut, Atlanta, Rural Georgia, Detroit, Iowa, Arizona, Hawaii, Los Angeles, New Mexico, San Francisco-Oakland, San Jose-Monterey, Seattle-Puget Sound and Utah). Those areas were chosen to represent the United States as a whole.

▸

Site

Location in the brain or spinal cord

▸ **WHO**

World **H**ealth **O**rganization

The author of the most widely used brain tumor classification system.

References

1. *CBTRUS (1999). Year 2000 Standard Statistical Report. Central Brain Tumor Registry of the United States, pages 7, 8, 14, 15, 17, 18.*

2. *Yung, A., Sawaya, R., Curran, W. and Fuller, G. "Intracranial Metastatic Central Nervous System Tumors," Cancer in the Nervous System. Churchill Livingstone, Inc., 1996, page 243.*

3. *Greenlee, R., Murray, T., Bolden, S., Wingo, P. "Cancer Statistics, 2000." January/February 2000. Vol. 50, No 1. CA: A Cancer Journal for Clinicians. American Cancer Society, pages 12, 13, 23.*

4. *Reis, LAG, Smith, MA, Gurney, JG (eds). Cancer Incidence and Survival among Children and Adolescents: United States SEER Program 1975-1995, National Cancer Institute, SEER Program, NIH Pub. No. 99-4649, 1999.*

Chapter 4

Causes

Many studies are underway to identify possible causes of primary brain tumors. Little is known, but researchers have begun to make progress. The more that is known, the more likely something can be done to prevent them.

Epidemiology is the study of the occurrence of a disease and the factors that influence it. Epidemiological studies gather information about who is affected. That data helps identify clusters of individuals who might be subject to common factors.

Laboratory studies investigate changes occurring on a cellular level that will lead to better understanding of the biological steps involved in tumor formation.

Areas of Investigation

Several genetic and environmental factors are being investigated.

▲ Genetic factors

It is generally accepted that a brain tumor is due to an alteration in the patient's genetic structure. The alteration can be inherited, caused by environmental factors, or a combination of the two.[1]

GENE ALTERATIONS

Scientists are focused on identifying the initial steps in the development of a brain tumor. It is theorized that multiple changes occur in a cell's DNA (genetic material) before a normal cell develops malignant potential. When a cell containing defective DNA multiplies, it produces two abnormal cells. Those abnormal cells continue to multiply, resulting in a tumor.

Laboratory studies are underway to catalog the genetic changes found in brain tumors and to seek the causes of those changes. Other research is investigating the processes that affect tumor cells, such as the production of growth factors—hormone-like substances produced by the body; angiogenesis—the process by which tumors increase their blood supply; and motility of tumor cells—movement away from the original tumor.

It is believed that altered (mutated) or missing genes enable cancer to develop. Proto-oncogene and tumor suppressor gene mutations are related to the development of cancer.

▸ Proto-oncogenes are normal genes that, when mutated, become oncogenes. If many oncogenes are present, a normal cell can be changed into a cancerous one.[2]

▸ Tumor suppressor genes deter cells from duplicating. If they are missing or altered, cells grow without interference.[2]

Both oncogenes and tumor suppressor genes are involved in the formation of a cancer.[2]

Researchers have identified several genetic abnormalities and related them to specific malignant brain tumors. For example, a gain of one or more copies of chromosome 7 is found in 80% of glioblastoma multiforme tumors; p53 mutation occurs 40-80% of the time.[1] Some genetic changes are unique to brain tumors; others occur with many types of cancer.[1]

HEREDITARY FACTORS

▸ Hereditary means inherited—transferred via genes from parent to child.

▸ Familial refers to the fact that two or more family members are affected, but it is not inherited.

Only about 5% of primary brain tumors are known to be associated with hereditary factors. In particular, those with Li-Fraumeni syndrome (LFS), p53 defects (usually associated with LFS), tuberous sclerosis, neurofibromatosis 1 and 2, von Hippel-Lindau disease, Turcot syndrome and familial polyposis have a higher incidence of brain tumors than the general population.

Families with higher-than-average cancer incidence may have an increased genetic pre-disposition, or it may be the result of exposure to the same environmental factors.[1]

▲ Environmental factors

Studies to identify possible environmental factors have examined three categories of agents [3]

▸ physical, such as electromagnetic fields

▸ chemical, such as N-nitroso compounds

▸ biological, such as viruses

PHYSICAL AGENTS

» **Low-frequency electromagnetic fields**
These low energy fields, called EMFs are emitted by power lines and household appliances. Low energy microwave frequencies are associated with cellular telephones.[3] This is an area of substantial research that has yielded no definitive results as yet.[3]

» **Ionizing radiation**
High-dose ionizing radiation, commonly used to treat brain tumors, has been related to second brain tumors in patients undergoing this form of treatment.[3]

Low-dose ionizing radiation, such as that emitted by diagnostic x-rays, is a minimal factor, if it all.[3] Past studies of exposure to ionizing radiation in the workplace have not found a correlation to brain tumors.[3]

CHEMICAL AGENTS

Brain tumors occur more frequently in people regularly exposed to: acrylonitrile, vinyl chloride, formaldehyde, lubricating oils, N-nitroso compounds, phenols, pesticides, polycyclic aromatic hydrocarbons and organic solvents.[3] Industries that could expose workers to those chemicals include: synthetic rubber and polyvinyl chloride manufacturers, crude oil and petroleum-based chemical producers, pharmaceutical manu-facturers, nuclear fuel and weapons producers and farms that use agricultural chemicals. Many workers are exposed to a combination of these agents.[3]

Researchers have just scratched the surface in their investigations into causal relationships. However, studies with animals indicate that the greatest risk of experiencing adverse effects of these chemicals is in utero or early infancy.[3]

BIOLOGICAL AGENTS

Exposure to viruses as a cause of brain tumors has been questioned. This area of investigation is underway.[3]

Prevention Research [4]

A large, coordinated study from eight centers in Europe, Israel and North America looked at a variety of factors that might affect the incidence of brain tumors in infants and children under the age of twenty. The study found that pregnant women who took vitamin supplements containing C, A, E and/or folate during the entire period of their pregnancy were half as likely to have their child develop a brain tumor before age 5, as compared to those who didn't take vitamins.

The antioxidant effects of vitamins C and E or the cell differentiation effects of vitamins A and D might be responsible for these results, or the vitamins might prevent the formation of other cancer-causing compounds in the body.

For More Information

To learn more about potential causes, you can perform a medical literature search on the Internet using **Medline** at **http://igm.nlm.nih.gov** Medline is a computer program that searches medical journals for articles containing the keywords and limits you specify. It has an easy "fill-in-the-blank" format and online help options.

Because Medline was designed for medical professionals, you must use medical terms as the keywords. For information on causes of brain tumors, use the terms *etiology* (cause) and *brain neoplasm* (brain tumor). If the program finds too many articles, you can add limits. For example, choose *review articles only*, or limit the search by entering additional keywords.

The search will list articles that meet your specifications. Some of the articles have abstracts and those may provide all the information you seek. Or you can ask a librarian to obtain the complete article for you.

If you don't have access to the Internet, some local libraries, many hospital libraries, and all university medical school libraries have access to Medline. Ask the reference librarian at your local library if they can provide access and what fees there might be for that service. Most medical school and hospital libraries will allow you to use their computer facilities. Call first to make sure they allow visitors.

Remember that the articles in Medline were written for a medical audience. If you have any questions about the information you find, your doctor is the best source for answers.

References

[1] Bondy, Wiencke, Wrensch, Kyritsis. "Genetics of primary brain tumors: a review." *Journal of Neuro-Oncology*. 18: 69-81, 1994.

[2] Wu, Haber. "Molecular Biology of Brain Tumors." *Neurosurgery Clinics of North America*. 5: 127-132, 1994.

[3] Thomas, Inskip. "Brain and Other Nervous System." *Cancer Rates and Risks, 4th Edition, 1996*. National Institutes of Health, National Cancer Institute.

[4] "Vitamins during Pregnancy Linked to Lower Risk of Childhood Brain Tumors." News. *Journal of the National Cancer Institute*. 89: 1481-1482, 1997.

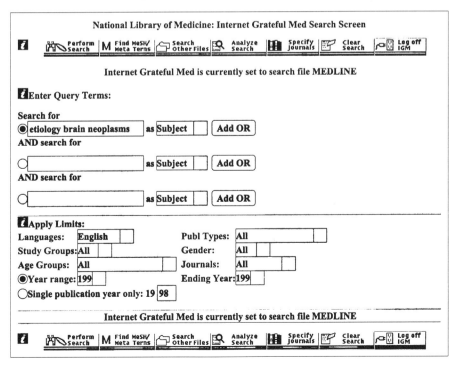

Chapter 5

Symptoms

Just as you are a unique individual, each brain tumor is unique also. General statements about symptoms can be made, but it might not be possible to predict exactly what your tumor will do. In this chapter, we hope to help you understand why symptoms occur by explaining the functions of the different parts of the brain.

Because symptoms are often vague and confusing, a brain tumor might be difficult to diagnose. Symptoms produced by a brain tumor often mimic the symptoms of other diseases and vice versa. Because symptoms can develop gradually, and because they can be subtle, it might be a long time between their onset and diagnosis.

General Symptoms

Some symptoms are due to increased pressure caused by the growing tumor. Other, more specific, symptoms are related to the tumor's location, type and size.

▲ Headaches

Headaches are a common initial symptom and the majority of patients experience headaches sometime during the course of their illness. Typical brain tumor headaches come and go and usually do not throb. They are worse in the morning and improve gradually during the day. They can rouse the person from sleep. These headaches can worsen with coughing, exercise, or with a change in position such as bending or kneeling.

Headaches are usually due to pressure in the brain. Some people experience neck pain as well.

▲ Seizures

Seizures are another common symptom of brain tumors. Seizures are caused by a disruption in the normal flow of electricity in the brain. Those sudden bursts of electricity can cause a variety of symptoms including convulsions, unusual sensations, and loss of consciousness. Focal seizures can also occur. Symptoms of a focal seizure depend upon the tumor's location and can include muscle twitching or jerking, abnormal smells or tastes, problems with speech or numbness and tingling.

Seizures are the presenting symptom in approximately one-third of patients. About half of all patients experience some form of seizure during their illness.

▲ Mental changes

Mental changes frequently occur. These can range from problems with memory, speech, communication and/or concentration to severe intellectual problems and confusion. Changes in behavior, temperament and personality are other indications of mental change.

Mental changes are caused directly by the tumor, by increased pressure within the skull or by involvement of the areas of the brain that control personality.

▲ Mass effect symptoms due to Increased IntraCranial Pressure (IICP)

IICP is caused by:

▸ the tumor's growth within the skull—an area enclosed by bone which cannot expand, and/or

▸ *hydrocephalus*—blockage of the fluid that flows around and through the brain, and/or

▸ *edema*—swelling of the brain around the tumor due to an accumulation of fluid.

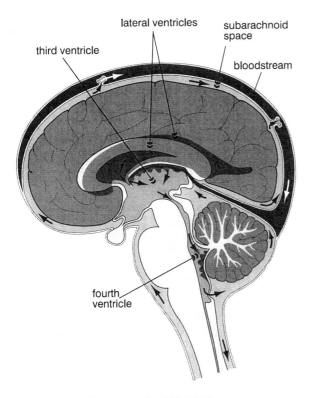

Cerebrospinal Fluid Flow

These all result in **mass effect**. Mass effect can cause further damage by compressing and displacing delicate brain tissue.

The symptoms caused by increased intracranial pressure include nausea and vomiting, drowsiness, vision problems such as blurred or double vision or loss of peripheral vision, and the headaches and mental changes already mentioned.

A swollen optic nerve *(papilledema)* is a clear sign of IICP. It can be observed by your doctor when he examines your eyes. This sign is common in young children, in persons with slow growing tumors, with tumors in the posterior fossa, and in older patients.

As pressure increases, the patient's level of consciousness decreases. Prompt treatment is required to avoid serious consequences.

▲ Focal Symptoms

In addition to the common, but non-specific symptoms listed above, other more specific symptoms frequently occur. These "focal symptoms" can help identify the location of the tumor. Focal symptoms include: hearing problems such as ringing or buzzing sounds or hearing loss, decreased muscle control, lack of coordination, decreased sensation, weakness or paralysis, difficulty with walking or speech, balance problems, or double vision.

Symptoms by Tumor Location

The following symptoms are due to a tumor's effect on specific brain structures. Symptoms might occur on the right side of the body if the tumor is located on the left side of the brain and vice-versa, depending on the specific brain structure affected.

BRAIN STEM TUMOR

Tumors of the Midbrain, Pons, Medulla Oblongata

The brain stem controls basic life functions including blood pressure, heart beat, and breathing. The reticular formation (the central core of the brain stem) controls consciousness, eating and sleeping patterns, drowsiness and attention.

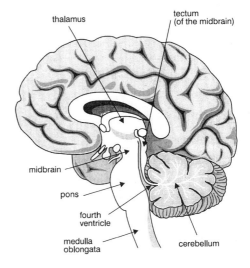

The Brain Stem

A tumor of the brain stem produces a variety of symptoms. The most common symptoms are vomiting (usually just after awakening), and a clumsy, uncoordinated walk. Muscle weakness on one side of the face causes a one-sided smile or drooping eyelid. Difficulty in swallowing and slurred or nasal speech are also common. In addition, double vision with an inability to fully move one or both eyes might occur. Headache, usually just after awakening, is common. Head tilt, drowsiness, hearing loss and/or personality changes can also be present. Symptoms may develop gradually.

CEREBELLUM TUMOR

Located in the posterior fossa, the cerebellum together with the thalamus and cerebrum controls intricate muscular coordination, including walking and speech. *See Posterior Fossa Tumor.*

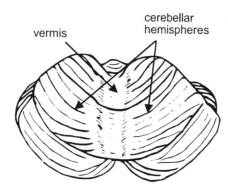

The vermis is involved with large movements of the entire body, and posture.

The hemispheres are involved with fine movements of the extremities (arms, legs, feet, hands).

The Cerebellum

CEREBELLOPONTINE ANGLE TUMOR

Usually an Acoustic Nerve Tumor

The earliest symptom is ringing or buzzing in the ear. Less often, dizziness might occur. As the tumor grows, deafness, loss of facial sensation and/or facial weakness can occur. Other symptoms are similar to those of a brain stem tumor.

CEREBRAL HEMISPHERE TUMOR

» **Frontal Lobe Tumor**

The frontal lobe of each hemisphere controls voluntary movement, usually on the opposite side of the body. The frontal lobe of the dominant hemisphere controls language and writing. (The dominant hemisphere is the left

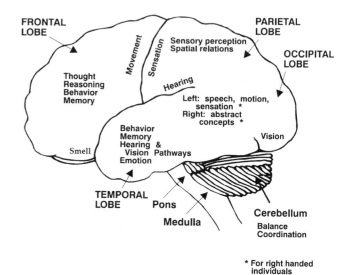

Lobes of the Brain

hemisphere in all right-handed and some left-handed individuals, and the right hemisphere in most left-handed people.) Other frontal lobe activities include intellectual functioning, thought processes, behavior, and memory.

Tumors in the frontal lobe may initially be "silent." As they grow, they can cause a variety of symptoms including one-sided paralysis, seizures, short-term memory loss, impaired judgment and personality or mental changes. Urinary frequency and urgency can develop. Gait disturbances and communication problems are also common.

If the tumor is at the base of the frontal lobe, loss of smell, impaired vision, and a swollen optic nerve can occur.

» **Occipital Lobe Tumor**

The occipital lobe is involved in the understanding of visual images and the meaning of written words.

Blindness in one direction or other visual disturbances, and seizures are common symptoms.

» **Parietal Lobe Tumor**

The parietal lobe receives and interprets sensations including pain, temperature, touch, pressure, size, shape, and body-part awareness. Other activities of the parietal lobe are hearing, reasoning and memory.

Seizures, language disturbances if the tumor is in the dominant hemisphere, and loss of ability to read are common symptoms. Spatial disorders, such as difficulty with body orientation in space or recognition of body parts, can also occur.

The parietal lobe also controls language and the ability to do arithmetic. Numbers may be read, but there may be difficulty with calculations. There may be difficulty knowing left from right and sentences containing comparisons or cross-references may not be understood.

» **Temporal Lobe Tumor**

The temporal lobe is involved in the understanding of sounds and spoken words, as well as emotion and memory. Depth perception and the sense of time are also controlled by the temporal lobe.

Seizures are the most common symptom of a tumor in this location. The ability to recognize sounds or the source of sounds may be affected. Vision can be impaired.

» **Basal Ganglia Tumor**

One-sided paralysis is the most common symptom. This tumor might invade other areas of the cerebral hemispheres and produce symptoms common to tumors in those locations. Seizures are uncommon.

» **Corpus Callosum Tumor**

Impaired judgment and defective memory are frequent symptoms of a tumor in the forward part of this area; behavioral changes are common with a tumor in the rear part. A tumor in the middle of the corpus callosum might cause few, if any, symptoms until it grows quite large.

This tumor might invade other lobes of the cerebral hemispheres and produce symptoms common to tumors in those locations. Seizures are uncommon.

FOURTH VENTRICLE TUMOR

See Posterior Fossa Tumor

HYPOTHALAMUS TUMOR

The hypothalamus controls thirst and urination, sleep, body temperature, appetite, and blood pressure. The hypothalamus coordinates patterns of activity and controls emotions. It is also the control center for the pituitary gland.

MEDULLA OBLONGATA TUMOR

The medulla oblongata, a part of the brain stem, controls swallowing, tongue movement, breathing, heart beat, and vomiting. *See Brain Stem Tumor.*

MENINGEAL BRAIN TUMOR

This type of tumor usually causes symptoms by pressure and compression rather than by growth into brain tissue. Seizures are common. Additional symptoms depend on the location of the tumor.

METASTATIC BRAIN TUMOR

Symptoms depend on the location of the tumor(s) in the brain or spine. Headache, nausea and vomiting are common due to the swelling that frequently accompanies these tumors. If the tumor is in the spine, pain might occur directly over the area of metastasis or radiate along the affected nerve.

MIDBRAIN TUMOR

The midbrain, a part of the brain stem, is a relay center for sight and hearing. Symptoms associated with this tumor usually involve the eye, such as eye movement disorders with double vision and abnormal pupil reactions. *See Brain Stem Tumor.*

MIDLINE TUMOR

The "midline" is where the two cerebral hemispheres meet. Headaches, nausea and a swollen optic nerve are the most common symptoms associated with this area and are due to increased intracranial pressure. Other symptoms are abnormal eye movements and vision, and alteration of personality or consciousness. In addition, impairment of glandular functions can cause either delayed or accelerated growth. The development of a water balance problem is possible.

OPTIC TRACT TUMOR

Symptoms associated with this tumor involve the eye and vision, such as eye movement disorders, abnormal pupil reactions and impaired vision. In addition, production of hormones can be affected due to the tumor's effect on the nearby pituitary. *See Midline Tumor.*

PINEAL TUMOR

A tumor in this location causes hydrocephalus with the symptoms of increased intracranial pressure. Problems with eye movement often occur. In children, hormonal disturbances such as precocious puberty may occur.

PITUITARY TUMOR

The pituitary is called the "master gland." It secretes several important hormones.

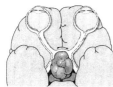
Pituitary tumor

Headache, vision changes, and diabetes insipidus (a type of hormone disturbance) are common symptoms. Because these tumors often secrete hormones inappropriately, other symptoms vary

depending on the type of hormone secreted. Breast enlargement and secretion are common.

PONS TUMOR

The pons, a part of the brain stem, coordinates the activities of the cerebrum and cerebellum by relaying impulses between them and the spinal cord.

Symptoms include weakness, loss of sensation, involuntary movements, abnormal eye movements, double vision, a clumsy uncoordinated walk, decreased facial sensation or movement, hearing loss and balance problems. *See Brain Stem Tumor.*

POSTERIOR FOSSA TUMOR

The posterior fossa contains the fourth ventricle, cerebellum and brain stem.

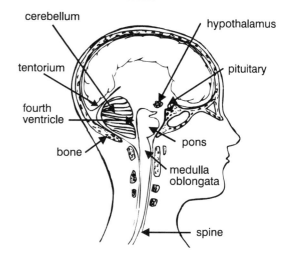

Headaches due to the tumor and/or hydrocephalus, nausea and vomiting, and a swollen optic nerve due to increased intracranial pressure are the most common symptoms. A clumsy, uncoordinated walk, swaying, and staggering might occur. Dizziness, tremors, as well as difficulty with coordination and speech, are also frequent symptoms. Double vision can occur. Nerve irritation can cause pain in the back of the head or neck or tilting of the head.

SELLAR, PARASELLAR TUMOR

The pituitary gland, hypothalamus and optic chiasm are in the sellar/parasellar region. Symptoms depend on the specific structure affected by the tumor.

SKULL BASE TUMOR

A wide variety of structures in the brain and head might be affected. Symptoms depend on the specific structure affected. Cranial nerves are often affected causing slurred speech, swallowing difficulties, double vision and facial weakness. Balance problems can occur.

SPINAL CORD TUMOR

Symptoms of these tumors depend on the nerves involved. A tumor of the thoracic area can cause a "girdle pain" in the chest that worsens with coughing or sneezing. This pain is often worse when the person is lying down. A tumor in the cervical or lumbar areas can cause neck, arm, back, or leg pain. Weakness, muscle wasting or spasms, and sensory changes are other common symptoms. Decrease or lack of bowel or bladder control can occur, depending on the location of the tumor.

THALAMIC TUMOR

The thalamus monitors input from the senses and acts as a relay station for the sensory center of the cerebrum.

Common symptoms include sensory loss such as the sense of touch on the side of the body opposite the side of the tumor; muscle weakness; decreased intellect; vision problems; speech difficulties; loss of urinary control; headache, nausea and vomiting and difficulties in walking due to the increased pressure caused by obstructive hydrocephalus.

THIRD VENTRICLE TUMOR

Hydrocephalus due to the blockage of cerebro-spinal fluid is very common, causing symptoms of increased intracranial pressure. Leg weakness, fainting spells, impaired memory and hypo-thalamic dysfunction are frequent symptoms. *See Hypothalamus Tumor.*

Chapter 6

Diagnosis and Follow-Up Testing

Initially, the question is whether or not you have a brain tumor. If you do, the next step is to determine the type of tumor.

Following treatment, some of the same tests used to first diagnose your tumor are repeated to monitor your progress—to see if the tumor has disappeared, is shrinking, remains the same or has changed. Follow-up care following diagnosis and treatment of a brain tumor might extend for years or even a lifetime, not unlike many other medical conditions.

Understanding the tests—what they are, how they work, and what they can or cannot show—can help you feel more comfortable and in control.

Your doctor begins to make a diagnosis by taking your medical history. You are asked to describe your symptoms, how long you have had them, when they occur, if they seem to be brought on by something in particular, the order of their appearance, and if they seem to be getting worse. Following the question and answer phase of the diagnosis, your doctor will perform a basic neurological examination.

Neurological Exam

A basic neurological examination includes the following:

- eye movement, pupil reaction, and eye reflex tests using a pen light, following a moving finger
- vision tests and examination of the optic nerve
- hearing tests using a ticking watch or tuning fork
- reflex tests using a rubber hammer
- balance and coordination tests—heel-to-toe walking, heel-to-shin movements; balance with feet together and eyes closed; rapid alternating movements such as touching the finger to the nose with eyes closed

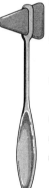

- sense of touch tests using a pin point and cotton ball
- sense of smell tests with various odors
- facial muscle tests—smiling, grimacing
- tongue movement, gag reflex tests
- head movement tests
- mental status tests—stating the current time and date, naming the current President
- abstract thinking tests—defining the meaning of "a stitch in time saves nine"
- memory tests—repeating a list of objects, describing the food you ate at yesterday's breakfast, what occurred last Thanksgiving

If the results of your neurological examination lead the doctor to suspect you have a brain tumor, a scan will be ordered, or you might be referred to a neurological specialist for additional testing. Those tests might include:

Scans

Scans take the place of conventional x-rays, which do not show tumors located behind the bones of the skull or spine. Different types of imaging devices are used to perform scans. The most common scans for diagnosis and follow-up are Computerized Tomography (CT) and Magnetic Resonance Imaging (MRI).

Both CTs and MRIs use computer graphics to create an image of the brain. An injection of a special contrast material (dye) to make abnormal tissue more obvious is usually given before the scan. The contrast materials concentrate in diseased tissues in greater quantity than in healthy tissues. That concentration is due to the leakiness of blood vessels in and around brain tumors. Contrast materials highlight abnormalities such as tumors.

Small tumors, tumors next to bone, brain stem tumors, low grade and metastatic tumors might be imaged better by the MRI than the CT. CT is more effective at showing calcification and bony erosion. Your doctor determines which scan/s to use.

▲ CT scan

This scan combines an x-ray device with a computer. For some types of tumors, CT images 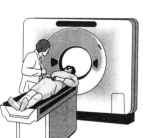 are obtained both with and without contrast enhancement to provide important additional information.

If contrast is used, it is usually injected after a few pictures are taken. The patient lies on a table that slides into a doughnut-shaped opening. The CT scanner circles the head so x-rays penetrate the brain from many directions. Absorption of the x-rays varies with the type of tissue penetrated. Thousands of thin cross-section readings are fed into the computer which transforms the information into a picture.

▲ MRI scan

The MRI is a tunnel-shaped piece of equipment. Some pictures are taken prior to contrast injection. If contrast is to be used, it is injected prior to the completion of the scan. The patient lies on a table that slides into the tunnel. Inside the scanner, a magnetic field surrounds the head. A radio frequency pulse is introduced to the area. No x-rays are used. The magnetic field causes atoms in the brain to change direction. The radio frequency pulse causes another change of direction. When the pulse stops, the atoms relax and return to their original position. During relaxation, the atoms give off energy in differing amounts and at different intervals of time. Antennas pick up these signals and feed them into a computer which assembles a picture. Because different atoms have their own characteristic radio signals, the computer can distinguish between healthy and diseased tissue.

Patients with cardiac monitors, pacemakers, or some types of surgical clips cannot undergo MRI scanning because of the magnetic fields. For those who are claustrophobic, sedation or "open" MRI scanners can be an option.

▲ Other CT or MRI based scans

Computer technology advances have made possible the development of new methods for using existing scanning equipment. These new methods provide advanced tools for diagnosis.

Most of these new tools measure the rate of blood flow into the brain. A contrast dye is given to the patient by intravenous (IV) infusion. The scanner begins taking pictures as soon as the dye is given. Using computerized timing, a succession of rapid pictures can be imaged, tracing the path of blood flow into the brain and to the brain tumor. These techniques are also used to scan spinal cord tumors.

These new methods are collectively called hemodynamic imaging. The information gathered can be converted into images or graphed into charts. Several different types of scanning equipment are used to produce these images: CT, MRI, PET, and SPECT.

DYNAMIC CT AND DYNAMIC MRI

The CT or MRI is combined with the ability to measure the uptake of the contrast dye from the time it begins to flow from the IV. Dynamic scans are especially useful in showing the growth of new blood vessels around a tumor.

FUNCTIONAL MRI (also called Echoplanar, "Real Time" or Fast MRI)

This technique produces MRI images in a faster sequence than traditional MRIs. The increased speed permits the tumor's use of oxygen to be depicted. This scan can be useful in distinguishing tumor from swelling (edema).

The speed at which images are produced makes functional MRI useful during surgery to show tumor bulk, or for brain mapping. Brain mapping helps the neurosurgeon determine, during surgery, the specific areas of the brain that control speech, movement, and memory so they can be avoided.

FLOW SENSITIVE MRI (FS MRI)

This type of scan combines functional MRI with images of cerebrospinal fluid (CSF) flow. FS MRI can be used to show the flow of CSF through the ventricles and spinal cord. It can be useful in planning for the surgical removal of a skull base tumor, spinal cord tumor, or a tumor causing hydrocephalus.

▲ Angiography and MRI Angiography (MRA)

Angiography is used to outline the presence and position of blood vessels in the brain. After injection of a contrast material into a deep artery, x-rays follow its flow through the blood vessels of the brain. MRI angiography, which is less invasive, uses a rapid succession of MRI scans to follow the blood flow.

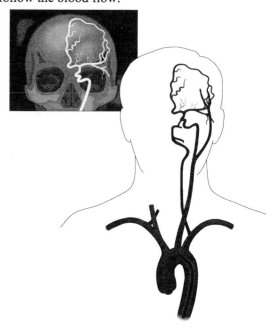

The role of angiography for brain tumors is usually limited to planning the surgical removal of a tumor suspected of having a large blood supply, or tumors growing into an area of the brain with an abundance of blood vessels.

▲ Holography

With Digital Holography, an exact replica of the internal structure of the body is obtained from CT or MRI slices. The holographic image is created by superimposing brightness and distance information of each slice and storing it on holographic film. The holographic image projects out into space. It is transparent and life-sized. Surgeons can place their instruments and tools inside the image just as if it were the "real thing." This planning and teaching tool is available at a small number of hospitals.

▲ MRS (Magnetic Resonance Spectroscopy)

MRS produces images depicting function rather than shape. The equipment requires a special, highly complex facility.

Capable of measuring some byproducts of living tissue (called metabolites), this non-invasive scanning technique can depict patterns of activity that may be useful in diagnosing specific tumors. The MRS may be useful with low grade gliomas, tumors with a large amount of surrounding edema and in differentiating between tumor recurrence and radiation necrosis. This technique may also be valuable in suggesting the degree of malignancy. MRS and PET are complementary tools for metabolic imaging.

▲ PET (Positron Emission Tomography)

PET is not routinely used for diagnosis but it can complement scanning information by suggesting tumor grade. It can also be used to try to distinguish between recurrent tumor versus cells killed by radiation (necrosis) versus scar tissue.

In a PET scan, a low-dose of radioactive sugar is injected into the patient. The PET scanner rotates around the patient's head, detecting the amount of radioactive sugar taken up by various parts of the brain. A growing tumor consumes glucose at a high rate; radiation necrosis or scar tissue consumes almost no sugar.

Measurements of brain activity (determined by concentrations of the glucose) feed into a computer, which produces a color-coded moving picture or a black and white image of the brain as it converts food (glucose) into energy.

The use of PET had been limited because it requires very scarce, complex equipment. There also can be false negatives and positives. An increasing number of facilities now have it available. A listing of PET sites is available from our office.

▲ SPECT (Single Photon Emission Tomography)

SPECT is not routinely used in the initial diagnosis of a brain tumor, but might complement information obtained from other scans.

A SPECT scan is similar to PET. Radioactive tagged materials taken up by the brain are used. A special camera measures the rate of emission of the material as it moves through the brain. Images are generated from that information.

After CT or MRI, this test might be helpful in distinguishing between low-grade and high-grade tumors, or between recurrent tumor and necrosis.

▲ MEG (Magnetoencephalography)

The MEG scan measures the magnetic fields created by nerve cells as they produce the small electrical currents used for neurotransmission. No physical contact is required to record the signals.

The device looks like an old-fashioned hair dryer. When the patient moves, a computer-generated image shows which brain area is responsible for directing the motion.

MEG is used in combination with information from other types of scans to determine the function of specific areas of the brain. Few MEG scanners are available.

X-Rays

Plain skull x-rays are usually not necessary for diagnosis except to help determine if calcification or bony erosion is present. Slow growing tumors can cause calcification; increased intracranial pressure might cause erosion. X-rays might be used to determine the condition of the skull adjacent to meningeal and skull base tumors.

A radiologist interprets the computer images produced by scans and x-rays. The pictures help establish a tentative diagnosis and might suggest the type of tumor—but they are not definitive. Only examination of a sample of tumor tissue under a microscope provides an exact diagnosis.

Laboratory Tests

▲ Lumbar puncture (Spinal tap)

Lumbar puncture is used to obtain a sample of cerebrospinal fluid (CSF). This procedure is usually avoided if there is any indication of increased intracranial pressure because of the risk of the brain's bulging through an opening in a membrane, muscle, or bone (herniation).

The sample of CSF is examined in a laboratory to determine if tumor cells, infection, protein, or blood is present. This information is particularly helpful in diagnosing primary CNS lymphoma, a pineal region or meningeal tumor. After surgery, the presence of tumor cells in the CSF indicates tumor spread. That information is used for tumor staging and helps the doctor determine appropriate treatment choices.

The CSF is also examined for the presence of known tumor markers, substances which indicate the presence of a tumor. Unfortunately, most primary brain tumors have no tumor markers. At this time, some germ cell tumors only are known to produce those substances. Known germ cell tumor markers are:

AFP   alpha-fetoprotein
HCG   human chorionic gonadotropin
PLAP   placental alkaline phosphatase

CEA (carcinoembryonic antigen) is a marker for a tumor of the arachnoid and/or pia mater membranes of the meninges (a leptomeningeal tumor). These are usually metastatic tumors.

If they are present, tumor markers are helpful in the diagnosis and follow-up evaluation of germ cell and metastatic brain tumors only.

▲ Myelogram

Lumbar puncture is used to inject a special dye before a myelogram. The patient is then tilted to allow the dye to mix with the spinal fluid. This test is used primarily to diagnose a spinal tumor and obtain pre-operative information for spinal tumor surgery.

Spinal MRI has replaced myelography for many conditions.

▲ Evoked-potentials

Evoked-potential testing uses small electrodes to measure the electrical activity of a nerve. This test is particularly useful in detecting an acoustic neuroma.

Evoked-potentials can also be used to monitor neurological function during the surgical removal of a tumor.

▲ Audiometry

This hearing test is useful in the diagnosis of a cerebellopontine angle tumor such as the acoustic neuroma.

▲ Endocrine evaluation

Measurements of hormone levels in samples of blood and urine are used, along with scans, to diagnose a pituitary or hypothalamic tumor.

▲ Perimetry

This technique measures the size of visual fields. The information obtained might be useful in diagnosing a tumor in the area of the optic chiasm, such as a pituitary tumor.

Biopsy

A biopsy is a surgical procedure in which a small amount of tumor tissue is removed. The neurosurgeon submits the tumor tissue to a pathologist for study and analysis. An exact diagnosis is then possible.

A biopsy can be performed as part of the surgery to remove the tumor, or as a separate diagnostic procedure.

For areas considered to be "inoperable," the surgeon is often able to perform a biopsy through a small hole drilled into the skull called a **burr hole**.

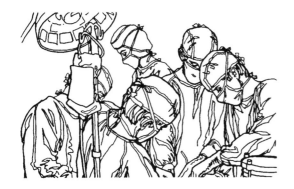

In a **needle biopsy**, a narrow, hollow needle is inserted through the burr hole. Tumor tissue is removed from the core of the needle.

Stereotaxic biopsy is a computer directed needle biopsy. The computer, using information from a CT or MRI scan, provides precise information about a tumor's location and its position relative to the many structures in the brain.

Stereotactically guided equipment might be moved into the burr hole to remove a sample of the tumor. This is called a **closed biopsy**.

When biopsy is not performed, diagnosis relies solely on the interpretation of other test results. *See also **Types of surgery** in Chapter 8.*

About Follow-Up Testing

At intervals during and after treatment, your doctor will probably order some of the same tests you took when your tumor was first diagnosed.

These tests measure the effectiveness of the treatment and monitor for possible recurrence. Other tests help evaluate your medication.

Your doctor will tell you when your next scans or tests should be done. If you don't have this information, **call your doctor's office and ask.** Follow-up is as important as treatment.

Chapter 7

Types of Brain and Spinal Cord Tumors

This chapter contains an **alphabetical** list of the more frequent brain and spinal cord tumors, their common locations, and how they might be treated. Please remember that **your** tumor is unique and might not conform to the "average" characteristics described.

The tumor names we use are based on the new WHO *(World Health Organization)* brain tumor classification system. If you cannot find a listing for your type of tumor, look at Appendix A, pages 114-116, or the index beginning on page 131.

Acoustic Neuroma
also called Neurilemmoma, Vestibular Schwannoma or Neurinoma

The acoustic neuroma is a benign tumor of the nerve of hearing (the 8th cranial nerve). It is located in the angle between the cerebellum and the pons, in the posterior fossa (the back of the skull). This tumor usually grows very slowly.

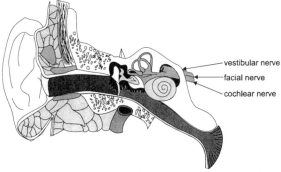

vestibular nerve
facial nerve
cochlear nerve

Cross section of the ear

Acoustic neuromas typically occur in adults, particularly in their middle years. Females are twice as likely to have this tumor as males. Acoustic neuromas account for fewer than 7.5% of all primary brain tumors.

Tumors on both sides (bilateral) are rare, and tend to be familial. They are almost always associated with *neurofibromatosis 2*, a hereditary condition. The malignant form of this tumor, **malignant peripheral nerve sheath tumor** (MPNST), is extremely rare.

Common symptoms are one-sided hearing loss and buzzing or ringing in the ear. Dizziness may also occur, but is less common. If the tumor also affects the facial nerve (the 7th cranial nerve) located next to the 8th nerve, facial paralysis can occur. Other symptoms include difficulty in swallowing, impaired eye movement, taste disturbances, and unsteadiness.

Total removal using microsurgical techniques is often possible. Stereotactic radiosurgery (see *Radiosurgery* in chapter 8) might be used as an alternate to surgery for some patients.

For more information about acoustic neuromas, contact the Acoustic Neuroma Association ▼ PO Box 12402 ▼ Atlanta, GA 30355 ▼ (404) 237-8023 ▼ Fax (404) 237-2704 ▼ E-mail ANAUSA@ aol.com ▼ http://www.ANAUSA.org

Astrocytoma

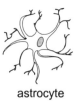

astrocyte

Astrocytomas are tumors that arise from astrocyte cells—part of the supportive (neuroglial) tissue of the brain. The cells are named for their star-like shape. Astrocytomas are the most common primary CNS tumors, representing about half of all primary brain and spinal cord tumors.

The major categories of astrocytoma are:
- *Pilocytic Astrocytoma* (WHO Grade I)
- *Astrocytoma* (WHO Grade II)
- *Anaplastic Astrocytoma* (WHO Grade III)
  (Separate publication available. See p. 137)
- *Glioblastoma Multiforme* (WHO Grade IV)
  (Separate publication available. See p. 137)

Other names for astrocytomas are based on their location, appearance or some other characteristic.
- **Glioma** is the generic name given to tumors arising from the supportive tissue of the brain (glia).
- **Brain stem glioma** is the generic name given to a tumor involving the brain stem when an exact diagnosis has not been determined.
- **Butterfly glioma** is a higher grade astrocytoma that has spread through both sides of the brain, causing a "butterfly" appearance on scans.
- **Cerebellar astrocytoma** *or* **cerebellar glioma** is the generic name given to a glial tumor of the cerebellum.
- **Mixed glioma** contains oligodendroglioma and/or ependymoma cells in addition to astrocytoma cells. Mixed gliomas are most commonly grade II or III tumors.
  (Separate publication available. See p 137.)

Astrocytoma (WHO Grade I)
▲ Pilocytic Astrocytoma
▲ Subependymal Giant Cell Astrocytoma

These are usually non-infiltrating tumors which occasionally form cysts or are enclosed in a cyst. Invasion or spread to other parts of the brain and spinal cord is rare. Although they are slow growing, these tumors can become very large.

Grade I tumors are often cured by surgery alone. Radiation therapy might follow surgery for incompletely removed tumors. If the tumor recurs, re-operation and some form of radiation are options. The value of chemotherapy and biologic response modifiers is being evaluated.

Pilocytic astrocytomas occur mainly in children. They are the most benign of the astrocytomas. Many **optic gliomas** and **cerebellar astrocytomas** are pilocytic astrocytomas. **Brain stem gliomas**, hemispheric and diencephalic gliomas can also be grade I tumors.

The **subependymal giant cell astrocytoma** is the ventricular tumor associated with tuberous sclerosis.

Astrocytoma (WHO Grade II)

The **fibrillary**, **gemistocytic** and **protoplasmic astrocytoma** and some **mixed gliomas** are grade II tumors. They are infiltrating tumors but grow relatively slowly. (There is some disagreement as to the grade of the gemistocytic astrocytoma. Some pathologists consider this to be a higher grade tumor.)

The **pleomorphic xanthoastrocytoma** most frequently occurs in the temporal lobe of children and young adults. It tends to spread locally into the adjacent meninges. Seizures are the most common symptom. This tumor is graded II-III.

The tumor's location may determine its treatment. Complete surgical removal is sometimes possible for accessible tumors, although these tumors can be locally invasive. If total surgical removal is achieved, periodic follow-up with MRI or CT scans might be the only additional care required.

Radiation therapy may be used in addition to surgery or for inoperable grade II astrocytomas. The role of chemotherapy in treating these tumors is under investigation. Further treatment might be recommended only if the tumor recurs. Intracavitary radiation might be effective for cystic tumors. Children younger than three might receive chemotherapy so that radiation can be delayed.

If the tumor recurs, re-operation and some form of radiation are options.

Astrocytoma (WHO Grade III)
▲ Anaplastic Astrocytoma
(Separate publication available. See page 137)

Anaplastic astrocytomas are infiltrating, malignant tumors. They grow more rapidly than lower grade tumors and often invade nearby, healthy tissue. These tumors recur more frequently and more quickly than lower grade tumors. Their tendency to spread into surrounding tissues makes it difficult to completely remove them during surgery. Some lower grade tumors might recur as higher grade tumors. **Brain stem gliomas**, **optic gliomas** and **cerebellar astrocytomas** can be grade III tumors.

Treatment recommendations are based on the location of the tumor, if and how far the tumor has spread, and the general health and age of the patient. Surgery plus radiation therapy or surgery plus radiation therapy and chemotherapy is the standard treatment for accessible grade III astrocytomas. Inoperable tumors are usually treated with radiation therapy. Chemotherapy might be recommended after surgery and/or radiation therapy. BCNU, a commonly used drug, or PCV—the combination of *procarbazine*, *CCNU* and *vincristine*—has shown promising results.

Many clinical trials are available for initial and recurrent tumors using various investigational forms of radiation, chemotherapy, biologic response therapy and gene therapy.

Astrocytoma (WHO Grade IV)
see Glioblastoma Multiforme

Astrocytoma, Cerebellar

More than 80% of the cerebellar astrocytomas are grade I, localized, cystic tumors although higher grades of tumor also occur. Malignant tumors and tumor spread are rare. The cerebellar location is more common in children than adults and is usually very accessible to the neurosurgeon.

Surgery is the primary treatment and if total removal is possible, additional therapy might not be needed. Many of the surgeries for grade I tumors achieve total removal. Radiation might be recommended for an incompletely removed or higher grade tumor, or further treatment might be needed only if the tumor recurs. For children under three, chemotherapy is often given so that radiation can be delayed.

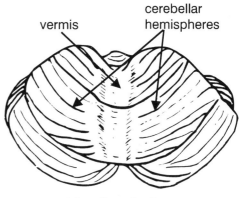

The Cerebellum

If the tumor recurs, a second surgery, radiation, or chemotherapy can be considered.

Atypical Teratoid/Rhabdoid Tumor (ATT/RhT)

This rare, high grade tumor occurs most commonly in children younger than two years of age. Its typical site is the cerebellum, and it frequently metastasizes throughout the central nervous system. These tumors are often confused with PNETs (primitive neuroectodermal tumors) or medulloblastoma, however the chromosome abnormalities are different. Treatment might include surgery, chemotherapy and radiation therapy.

Chondroma

This rare, benign tumor tends to arise at the base of the skull, especially in the area near the pituitary gland. It is very slow growing and might be present for a long time before causing any symptoms.

The chondroma is composed of cartilage formed by the meninges and is usually attached to the dura mater, the outermost layer of the meninges. It can grow to a large size, and can occur as single or multiple tumors. The malignant form of this tumor is the **chondrosarcoma**.

Because it is usually accessible with well-defined margins, surgery might be the sole treatment required for the chondroma.

Chondrosarcoma

This very rare tumor arises from bone and is composed of cartilage. It is the malignant variant of the benign chondroma and is a locally invasive tumor. This tumor rarely metastasizes, and is relatively slow growing. Its most common site is the sphenoid bone or clivus, at the base of the skull. The chondrosarcoma is more common in male adults.

Standard treatment is surgical removal which might be followed with radiation therapy. Clinical trials are also available.

Chordoma

The chordoma occurs at the base of the skull in about one third of patients, or at the end of the spine. It is a benign, slow growing, extradural tumor. However, it often invades adjacent bone and might compress the brainstem or grow into the sinuses. Distant spread is rare. This uncommon tumor represents 0.2% of all primary CNS tumors. The chordoma occurs in people of all ages, but is most frequent in younger and middle-aged adults.

The most common symptoms are double vision and headache.

The chordoma is visible on CT and MRI scans, but a biopsy is necessary to determine an exact diagnosis. The skull base location is very difficult to access.

Complete surgical resection might be possible for the spinal chordoma. A combination of surgery followed by radiation is the standard treatment for tumors located in the skull base. Stereotactic radiosurgery and stereotactic radiotherapy have shown promise, as have the combination of radical surgery followed by combined proton-photon beam therapy.

Choroid Plexus Carcinoma

This tumor, which occurs primarily in children, is the malignant form of the choroid plexus papilloma. It comprises about ten percent of all choroid plexus tumors and typically occurs in one of the lateral ventricles. (The choroid plexus carcinoma is sometimes called an **anaplastic choroid plexus papilloma**.) These tumors commonly invade adjacent tissue and spread widely via the cerebrospinal fluid. Hydrocephalus is often present.

Treatment often includes surgery, chemotherapy and radiation therapy. A second surgery might be recommended for recurrent tumors, followed by some form of radiation and/or chemotherapy.

Choroid Plexus Papilloma

The choroid plexus papilloma is a rare, benign tumor most common in children under the age of two. About 3% of the primary brain tumors in children are choroid plexus papillomas. They represent fewer than 1% of all primary brain tumors. The *choroid plexus carcinoma* is the malignant form of this tumor.

In very young children, the lateral ventricles are the most common location of this tumor. The fourth ventricle is the most common site in adults. Both CT and MRI scans detect these tumors.

The choroid plexus papilloma grows slowly within the ventricles. It eventually blocks the flow of cerebrospinal fluid, causing hydrocephalus and increased intracranial pressure. Headache and other symptoms of increased pressure are common.

The standard treatment is surgery and may be the only treatment required if the tumor is completely removed. Tumor removal relieves the hydrocephalus about half the time. A shunt is required for the other patients. The role of radiation or chemotherapy is still being investigated, but might be recommended for inaccessible or partially resected tumors.

Craniopharyngioma

This is a benign tumor arising from small nests of cells located near the pituitary stalk. Craniopharyngiomas represent 2-3% of all primary brain tumors, and 5-13% of childhood brain tumors. About sixty percent of craniopharyngiomas occur in patients older than sixteen.

Adamantinomatous (ordinary) craniopharyngioma occurs in children and tends to be more cystic than the **papillary** craniopharyngioma. The papillary craniopharyngioma occurs in adults and is a more solid tumor.

Craniopharyngiomas occur in the sellar region, near the pituitary gland. They often involve the third ventricle, optic nerve, and pituitary gland. These localized tumors grow by expansion and may reach a large size before they are diagnosed. Malignancy and metastasis are unknown.

Increased intracranial pressure due to obstruction of the foramen of Monro, one of the small tunnels through which cerebrospinal fluid exits the ventricles, accounts for many of the symptoms associated with this tumor. Other symptoms result from pressure on the optic tract and pituitary gland. Obesity, delayed development, impaired vision, and a swollen optic nerve are common.

Surgery and/or radiation therapy are the standard treatments and may be the only treatment/s needed if the tumor is completely removed. Radiation therapy for an incompletely removed tumor might be recommended. Intracavitary radiation or stereotactic radiosurgery might be used as forms of local therapy. Hormone therapy may be advised. In children younger than three, radiation is delayed if possible.

Cyst

Cysts are tumor-like spheres filled with fluid, similar to a balloon filled with water.

Cyst, Arachnoid

An arachnoid cyst (sometimes called a **leptomeningeal cyst**) is an enlarged, fluid-filled area of the subarachnoid space—the space between the arachnoid and pia mater layers of the meninges. It can occur in both adults and children. This cyst's most common locations are in the area of the Sylvian fissure, the cerebellopontine angle, the cisterna magna or the suprasellar region (see diagrams of the brain in Chapter 1, pages 9-14). The usual treatment is surgery to drain and remove the cyst's lining. Shunting may be required.

Cyst, Colloid

The third ventricle (see diagram, page 12) is the most frequent location of the benign colloid cyst. Malignant forms are unknown. This cyst almost always occurs in adults. It is typically attached to the roof of the third ventricle and the choroid plexus. This location commonly obstructs the foramen of Monro, one of the small tunnels through which cerebrospinal fluid exits the ventricles, causing increased intracranial pressure. Headache is the most common symptom.

Various surgical approaches, stereotactic directed cyst drainage or shunting are some of the treatment options for the colloid cyst. Removing this cyst without causing undue damage is very difficult, and the "best" treatment is still under discussion and study.

Cyst, Dermoid

A dermoid cyst is a distinct mass and is almost always benign. The standard treatment is surgical removal. If it returns, growth is very slow.

This cyst is more common in the spine than in the brain. The incidence in the brain is greatest in children under the age of ten. The lower end of the spine is the more common location in young people between the ages of 10 and 20.

A dermoid cyst in the brain is usually located at the midline of the cerebellum in the lower back portion of the brain, or the adjacent meninges. The cavity of the fourth ventricle and the base of the brain under the surface of the frontal lobes are also common sites (see diagrams, pages 9 and 10).

Cyst, Epidermoid

This type of cyst is more common than the dermoid. It is usually benign, but will slowly recur if not removed completely. Unlike the dermoid variety, an epidermoid cyst occurs more frequently in the brain than in the spine.

Epidermoid cysts are most common in middle-aged adults. Its most frequent locations are the cerebellopontine angle and the pituitary area.

The standard treatment is surgical removal.

Dysembryoplastic Neuroepithelial Tumor (DNT)

This tumor is similar in behavior to the oligodendroglioma. Although it occurs in both adults and children, the average patient with this grade I,

slow-growing tumor is under the age of twenty, and has a history of uncontrollable seizures of the partial complex type.

The DNT is most commonly located in a temporal or frontal lobe of the cerebrum. (See the diagram on page 10.) DNT is usually diagnosed following a long history of seizures.

Surgery alone often results in long term control for this tumor. The benefit of radiotherapy is yet to be determined.

Ependymoma

(Separate publication available. See page 137)

An ependymoma arises from the ependymal cells that line the ventricles and central canal of the spinal cord. (See diagram on page 12.) Ependymomas represent about 6% of all gliomas, and 10% of all childhood brain tumors. About 65% of ependymomas occur in the posterior fossa, the lower back portion of the brain. The remainder are found higher in the brain or in the spinal cord. Ependymomas are more common in children, but they also occur in adults.

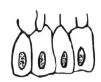
ependymal cells

About 10% of these tumors, particularly those of higher grade, spread via the cerebrospinal fluid (CSF). A spinal MRI with gadolinium enhancement can often detect if spread has occurred. A spinal tap is performed to test the CSF for the presence of tumor cells.

There are two types of grade I, benign ependymomas: **myxopapillary ependymoma** commonly found in the spine; and **subependymoma**. The subependymoma most often arises in the 4th ventricle; the second most frequent location is one of the lateral ventricles. The grade I tumors might be treated by surgery alone if the tumor is totally removed. Radiation therapy may be recommended following surgery if any tumor remains.

The **papillary, cellular,** and **clear cell ependymomas** are grade II tumors. These tumors are most frequently located in the fourth ventricle and the midline area. The extremely rare **papillary ependymoma** is located in the cerebellopontine angle. **Anaplastic ependymoma** is the grade III, malignant form of this tumor, and its typical location is the cerebral hemispheres. The rare **ependymoblastoma**, a high-grade, grade IV tumor, is more common in children and is classified as a PNET (primitive neuroectodermal tumor) in some systems.

An ependymoma can also be classified as "low-risk" or "high-risk," based on the location of the tumor and if tumor cells are found in the cerebrospinal fluid. Tumors in the fourth ventricle and midline are often more difficult for the neurosurgeon to access than those located in the cerebral ventricles.

The usual treatment for the higher grade tumors is surgery followed by radiation therapy to the brain and spinal cord. A shunt is often necessary to relieve the increased intracranial pressure that frequently accompanies this tumor. Chemotherapy or a form of local radiation might be used for recurrent tumors. Clinical trials using chemotherapy for initial treatment along with surgery and radiation are available. In very young children (under the age of three), chemotherapy might be used to delay radiation.

Gangliocytoma
Ganglioglioma

These rare, benign tumors arise from ganglia-type cells, which are groups of nerve cells. Gangliocytomas (sometimes called **ganglioneuromas**) are tumors of mature ganglion cells. Gangliogliomas are tumors of both mature nerve and supportive cells.

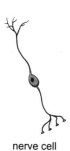
nerve cell

Tumors arising from ganglia most frequently occur in children and young adults. They represent 0.4% of all primary brain tumors and about 4% of all pediatric brain tumors.

The most common sites are the temporal lobe of the cerebral hemispheres and the third ventricle, although they might also occur in the spine. Cyst formation and calcification can be present. Seizures are the most common symptom.

These tumors are small, slow growing, and have distinct margins. Metastasis and malignancy are very rare.

Surgery is the standard treatment.

Germ Cell Tumors

These uncommon tumors represent 1 – 3% of childhood brain tumors and occur primarily in young people between the ages of 11 and 30. Germ cell tumors arise in the pineal or suprasellar regions of the brain. Included in this type of tumor are the **germinoma**, the **teratoma**, the more aggressive **embryonal carcinoma** and **yolk sac** (**endodermal sinus**) tumors, and the **choriocarcinoma**. Mixed germ cell tumors also exist. Because all these tumors tend to spread via the cerebrospinal fluid (CSF), diagnosis includes evaluation of the entire brain and spinal cord. An MRI scan with gadolinium enhancement and examination of the CSF for the presence of tumor cells is used for that evaluation.

Germ cell tumors are the only primary brain tumors that might be diagnosed by tumor markers found in the cerebrospinal fluid and blood. The markers are alpha-fetoprotein (AFP), placental alkaline phosphatase (PAP) and human chorionic gonadotropin (HCG). More commonly, however, the markers are used to monitor the effectiveness of therapy and to detect recurrence.

Because of its location, a germ cell tumor is often treated with chemotherapy or a combination of radiation and chemotherapy rather than surgery, although a biopsy to establish an exact diagnosis is not uncommon.

Germinoma

The germinoma is the most common type of **germ cell tumor** in the brain. It typically occurs in the pineal or suprasellar region of the brain. Because it tends to spread via the cerebrospinal fluid, diagnosis includes evaluation of the entire brain and spinal cord. An MRI scan with gadolinium enhancement and examination of the CSF for the presence of tumor cells is used for that evaluation.

The germinoma is the most frequent tumor of the pineal region (see the diagram on page 14) representing one-third of those tumors. It most commonly occurs in teen-aged children, and in males more often than females.

Tumors in the pineal region typically cause symptoms indicating increased intracranial pressure, and vision changes. Headache due to obstructed cerebrospinal fluid flow is the most common symptom. If the tumor is in the suprasellar location, symptoms include diabetes insipidus, vision changes and signs of hormonal dysfunction, such as fatigue, poor appetite, vomiting, delayed or absent puberty, changes in the menstrual cycle.

Surgery for germinoma depends on its accessibility and position relative to critical brain structures. The germinoma is very responsive to radiation and this can be an effective treatment for some patients. Chemotherapy might be the treatment of choice for some newly diagnosed tumors. Chemotherapy can also be useful for recurrent tumors.

Glioblastoma Multiforme (GBM)

(Separate publication available. See page 137)

The grade IV group of astrocytomas is represented by the Glioblastoma Multiforme and its variants, **gliosarcoma** and **giant cell glioblastoma**. These are all malignant tumors which commonly invade adjacent tissue and spread throughout the CNS. Fast growing astrocytomas that contain areas of dead tumor cells *(necrosis)* are classified as glioblastomas. GBMs most frequently arise in the white matter of the frontal lobes of the cerebral hemispheres (see the diagram on page 10).

GBM represents about 30% of all primary brain tumors and about 50% of the astrocytomas. It is more common in older adults, and affects more men than women. Nine percent of childhood brain tumors are glioblastomas.

Because the GBM grows very fast, the first symptoms are usually due to increased pressure in the brain. Headaches, seizures, memory loss, and changes in behavior are the most common presenting symptoms.

While many tumors contain a mixture of cell types, GBM is the most mixed of brain tumors. It is this characteristic that makes it one of the most difficult brain tumors to treat. While one cell type is responsive to treatment and dies off, other types wait for their chance to take over.

The first procedure for a GBM, if it is accessible, is surgery. If surgery is not an option, a biopsy might be recommended to confirm the type of tumor. Surgery alone rarely controls the GBM however, because cells of the tumor stray into other areas of the brain. Thus, radiation therapy almost always follows surgery or biopsy. Conventional external beam radiation might be used with a "boost" of local radiation, such as stereotactic radiosurgery or interstitial radiation (see pages 63 – 65). Other forms of radiation therapy for GBM are available.

Chemotherapy might be given before, during or after radiation. The most commonly used drugs for adults are BCNU, CCNU and procarbazine. Chemotherapy might be used in children under the age of three to delay radiation.

Recurrent tumors can be treated with additional surgery, chemotherapy and/or radiation therapy. Although conventional external beam radiation can only be received once, several newer forms of radiation therapy can follow standard treatment.

Many clinical trials are underway using gene therapy, monoclonal antibodies, biologic response modifiers, and chemotherapeutic agents. Radiation sensitizers, chemotherapy sensitizers, boron neutron capture therapy, photodynamic therapy, immunotoxins, differentiating agents, antisense drugs and antiangiogenic drugs are also being investigated (see Chapter 8, *Treatment*).

Glioma

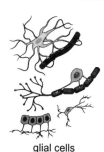

glial cells

This is a general name for tumors that arise from the supportive tissue (called glial or neuroglial tissue) of the brain. Gliomas are the most common primary brain tumors. Astrocytomas, ependymomas, oligodendrogliomas, and tumors with mixtures of two or more of these cell types are the most common gliomas.

Names such as **optic tract glioma** and **brain stem glioma** indicate the location of the tumor and are used when a specific diagnosis is not available. If a sample of the tumor is obtained during surgery or biopsy, a specific diagnosis is possible.

Glioma, Brain Stem

A brain stem glioma arises in or on the midbrain, pons, medulla oblongata, tectum, cervico-medullary junction or the dorsum (back) of the brain stem. Between 10 and 20% of brain tumors in children are brain stem gliomas. The tumor might be any type of astrocytoma, a ganglioglioma or an ependymoma. In patients for whom a biopsy is not possible, the specific type of tumor might not be known. These tumors do not commonly spread beyond the brain stem.

There are four groups of brain stem gliomas:
  ▶ *Diffuse*
  ▶ *Focal*
  ▶ *Exophytic*
  ▶ *Cervicomedullary*

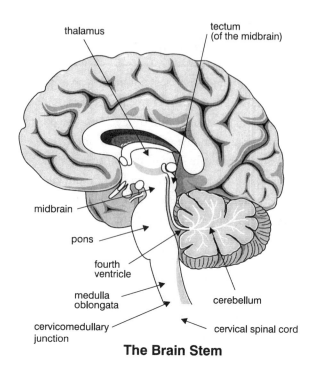

The Brain Stem

About 60-70% of brain stem tumors are **diffuse** (invasive or poorly delineated). These tumors have a rapid onset of symptoms. MRI scans show areas of tumor within the pons or medulla, and some tumors extend into the thalamus and upper cervical spine as well. The majority of these tumors are **fibrillary** or **anaplastic** gliomas.

Ten to twenty percent of brain stem gliomas are **focal** (confined to one area). They can be solid or cystic, and can occur in any part of the brain stem. **Tectal gliomas** located at the back of the midbrain are solid, focal, often slow-growing tumors. Focal tumors usually have a gradual onset of symptoms, and have the most optimistic prognosis. They are often **pilocytic** or **fibrillary** astrocytomas, and may be treated surgically.

An **exophytic** tumor arises in the brain stem, but often grows outward into the fourth ventricle. The symptoms are usually due to increased intracranial pressure caused by blockage of the flow of fluid from the ventricle.

A **cervicomedullary** tumor arises in the medulla oblongata and extends into the cervical spinal cord. It is often a **pilocytic** or **fibrillary astrocytoma**, and may be treated surgically.

Treatment for a brain stem glioma is dictated by the location and grade of the tumor. Micro-surgery, stereotactic surgery or imaging, evoked potentials and brain mapping might allow for biopsy or partial removal of focal, exophytic, or cervicomedullary tumors. Pre-surgical planning takes into account the surgical risks, as well as the type of tumor. Some brain stem gliomas, such as tectal gliomas and pilocytic astrocytomas might require no immediate therapy beyond repeat MRI scans and treatment of any existing hydrocephalus.

Radiation therapy, including hyperfractiona-tion, might be used as a primary treatment for inoperable or malignant tumors. It may also follow surgery for a partially removed tumor. Stereotactic radiosurgery might be used as a local form of radiation.

Chemotherapy might be recommended for patients with recurrent tumors. Children younger than three may be given chemotherapy to delay radiation. Clinical trials using various forms and schedules of radiation therapy, and chemotherapy for a recurrent tumor are available.

Glioma, Mixed

▲ **Oligo-Astrocytoma**

▲ **Anaplastic Oligo-Astrocytoma**

(Separate publication available. See page 137)

These tumors contain a high proportion of more than one type of cell. Mixed gliomas commonly contain both astrocytes and oligodendrocytes. Occasionally, ependymal cells are also found.

The behavior of these tumors is similar to tumors composed of the highest grade of cell present.

Standard treatment for a mixed glioma is the same as for an astrocytoma or oligodendroglioma of the same grade: surgery, often followed by radiation therapy. Chemotherapy might be used depending on the type of cells found in the tumor. Since oligodendrogliomas appear to respond well to chemotherapy, treatment with the drug combination PCV *(procarbazine, CCNU, vincristine)*

might be used. There are many clinical trials open to patients with mixed gliomas.

Glioma, Optic

These tumors may involve the optic chiasm, the optic nerve and the optic tract. They might affect the optic nerve alone, or extend along the visual pathway. This tumor does not spread to other areas of the brain. Optic gliomas most often occur in children under the age of 10. The grade I **pilocytic astrocytoma** and grade II **fibrillary astrocytoma** are the most common tumors in this area. Higher grade tumors may also arise in this location.

Twenty percent of children with **neuro-fibromatosis 1** will develop an optic glioma, typically a grade I, pilocytic astrocytoma. Children with optic gliomas are usually screened for neuro-fibromatosis (NF) for this reason.

The symptoms of a tumor in this area include loss of vision, rapid movement of the eyeballs and "crossed eyes." Hormonal disruption might also occur, causing developmental delay and other like symptoms.

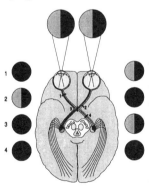

Careful observation only may be a treatment option for children with NF or slow growing tumors. Surgery might be recommended for a growing tumor involv-ing only the optic nerve. Radiation therapy might be used for a tumor of the chiasm or pathway. Local radiation therapy or chemotherapy with radiation therapy is used for recurrent tumors. Clinical trials are available for both primary and recurrent tumors.

Gliomatosis Cerebri

This condition is similar to glioblastoma multi-forme, but the cells of gliomatosis cerebri are more scattered and widespread. It also lacks the necrotic center of GBM. The diffuse nature of gliomatosis causes enlargement of the cerebrum, cerebellum or brain stem. Symptoms are often nonspecific, and can include personality changes, memory disturbance and seizures. Treatment is similar to that used for a glioblastoma multiforme.

Glomus Jugulare

Glomus jugulare tumors are very rare, slow growing, and benign. They widely invade the temporal bone. It is the most common tumor of the middle ear. Glomus jugulare tumors occur most often in women in their 50s.

Its location in the jugular foramen at the base of the skull causes symptoms that include hoarseness, swallowing difficulties, hearing loss or a ringing in the ear. Dizziness or blackouts might occur.

Initial diagnosis can be made with CT or MRI scanning. Confirmation can be made with cerebral angiography because this tumor often has a large blood supply. Multiple tumors are associated with genetic disorders.

The most effective treatment for this tumor is under debate. Radiation, radiosurgery, surgery or a combination of these might be appropriate. The surgical team often consists of a neurosurgeon and a head and neck surgeon. For those tumors which cannot be totally removed by surgery, or when surgery is not possible, radiation therapy or radiosurgery may be recommended.

Hemangioblastoma

This benign, tumor-like mass arises from blood vessels and is often cystic. Single or multiple tumors may be present. Hemangioblastomas represents about 2% of all primary brain tumors. **Lindau disease** or **von Hippel-Lindau disease** is an inherited condition which predisposes to this tumor and kidney cancer.

Hemangioblastoma is most frequent in the 35 to 45 age group. The most common site is the cerebellum. It is slow growing and does not spread.

This tumor commonly causes increased intracranial pressure and cerebellar dysfunction. Symptoms include headache, nausea and vomiting, gait disturbances, and balance problems.

CT or MRI scans can be used to detect the hemangioblastoma. Angiography is done before surgery to confirm the diagnosis and provide information about the tumor's blood supply.

Surgery is the standard treatment. Incompletely removed tumors or tumors attached to the brain stem might be treated with radiation therapy.

For more information about von Hippel-Lindau disease, contact the von Hippel-Lindau Family Alliance ▼ 171 Clinton Road ▼ Brookline, MA 02146 ▼ (800) 767-4845 ▼ Fax (617) 734-8233 ▼ E-mail vhl@vhl.org ▼ http://www.vhl.org

Hemangiopericytoma

This is a rare, grade II or grade III tumor, different from the meningioma although arising from the same cells. It is attached to the dura mater (the outermost layer of the meninges) and does not usually invade the brain itself. The hemangiopericytoma represents far less than 1% of all primary brain tumors. It most commonly occurs in men ages 38 to 42, in the lower back portion of the brain (posterior fossa) or in the spine.

These tumors frequently recur and tend to spread both within and outside the brain. Common sites of spread include bone, the lungs and the liver.

Standard treatment is surgery followed by radiation therapy. More than 50% of the time, the tumor can be totally removed. Long term follow-up with chest x-rays and liver function studies is necessary.

Lipoma

Lipomas are rare, benign tumors composed of fat tissue. The most common location is in the corpus callosum, but they also occur in many other areas in the brain. A lipoma might cause no symptoms and is often diagnosed coincidentally when scans are performed for other medical reasons. The most common symptom is seizures. It can be diagnosed by either CT or MRI scanning. Conservative treatment may include shunting to relieve pressure in the brain. The possibility of surgery depends on the tumor's position.

Lymphoma

also called CNS Lymphoma
Primary Malignant Lymphoma *or*
Primary CNS Lymphoma (PCL)

This disease affects people with healthy immune systems *and* those whose immune system is not functioning properly. People with malfunctioning immune systems include those who have undergone organ transplants or those infected with the AIDS virus. This lymphoma is most commonly B-cell, non-Hodgkin's type. The incidence of CNS lymphoma is increasing in people with healthy or unhealthy immune systems.

The most common sites of the lymphoma are the cerebral hemispheres. Multiple tumors can be present and spread throughout the central nervous system is common. Lymphomas appear on CT and MRI, but exact diagnosis requires a biopsy. A spinal tap to screen for tumor cells might be performed if there is no indication of increased intracranial pressure. Examination of other parts of the body is often recommended to determine if there is spread.

Symptoms include those associated with increased intracranial pressure, confusion, lethargy, mental changes, memory loss, muscle weakness in one area of the body, and seizures. Vision problems may be the first indication of the tumor.

Surgery or biopsy for diagnosis is usually performed. After the diagnosis of lymphoma has been confirmed, steroids are used to control brain swelling, and might result in the immediate disappearance of the tumor on a subsequent scan. Radiation therapy has been the standard therapy as these tumors respond well to radiation. Because this tumor often infiltrates large areas, the entire brain might be radiated. Chemotherapy used before and after radiation or in place of radiation might provide the greatest control.

Blood brain barrier disruption before chemotherapy using high dose intravenous methotrexate, and intraventricular methotrexate before radiation therapy are being investigated. Other chemotherapy clinical trials are available.

Medulloblastoma (MDL)

(Separate publication available. See page 137)

Medulloblastoma represents 15-20% of pediatric brain tumors. In addition, 30% of these tumors occur in adults. The MDL is always located in the cerebellum.

Medulloblastoma is a fast-growing, invasive tumor which frequently spreads to other parts of the central nervous system via the spinal fluid. This tumor can infiltrate the floor of the fourth ventricle and extend into its cavity. It can also infiltrate the meninges. The medulloblastoma can spread outside the brain and spinal cord, although this is uncommon.

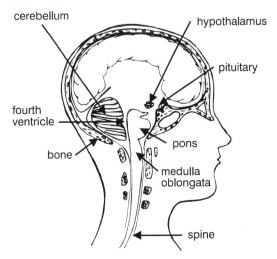

Treatment consists of surgical removal of as much tumor as possible, followed by staging. For children over the age of three and adults, radiation to the tumor area followed by a lower dose to the entire brain and spinal cord follows surgery. Very young children are often treated with chemotherapy instead of radiation until they are older. This tumor is very responsive to treatment with surgery, radiation and chemotherapy. Many clinical trials are available using chemotherapy.

"High-risk patients"— children younger than three, those with residual tumor following surgery, evidence of metastases, or with tumors involving the brain stem—usually receive chemotherapy, such as vincristine, CCNU and/or cisplatin as part of their initial treatment. Standard-risk patients treated with chemotherapy might receive lower doses of radiation. Recurrent tumors might require a second surgery followed by chemotherapy.

Meningioma

(Separate publication available. See page 137)

These tumors arise from the arachnoid cells of the meninges of the brain and spinal cord. They represent about 20% of all primary brain tumors and occur most commonly in middle-aged women.

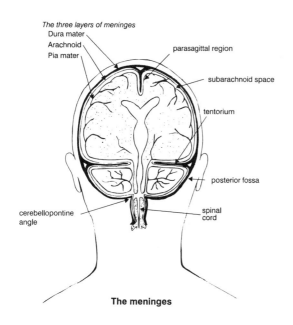

The meninges

Although the majority of meningiomas are benign, they can recur, sometimes as a higher grade tumor. Frequent sites are the parasagittal region, the posterior fossa, the cerebellopontine angle, and the base of the skull. Approximately fifty percent of the meningiomas occur in the parasagittal location. They less commonly occur in the spine, yet represent 25% of all primary tumors in that location. Meningiomas can be associated with **neurofibromatosis 2** or with prior radiation of the head or brain. They are most often single, but multiple tumors also occur.

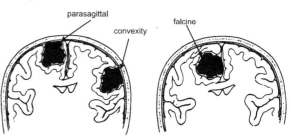

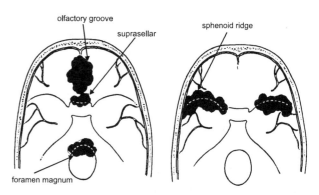

Common locations of meningiomas

A variety of symptoms are possible, depending on the tumor's location. The most common indications are headache, muscle weakness, seizures, personality change, confusion and visual impairment. In children, initial symptoms may be those indicating increased intracranial pressure.

The **benign meningioma** is slow growing with distinct borders. Because it is slow growing, it can grow quite large before symptoms become obvious. Symptoms are caused by compression rather than by invasion of brain tissue. If the tumor is accessible, the standard treatment is surgery to remove the tumor, the portion of the dura to which it is attached and any bone that is involved.

Radiation therapy or radiosurgery might be of value if the tumor is not entirely resected. Hormone therapy is under investigation. For some patients, surgery may not be recommended. For those with no symptoms (when they have been diagnosed coincidentally), those with minor symptoms of long duration and those for whom surgery would be risky, long-term close observation may be advised.

The **atypical meningioma** has a middle range of behavior. These tumors are not clearly malignant, but they may invade and spread within the brain, have a tendency to recur and are faster growing. This diagnosis is determined by specific features that can be seen under the microscope.

Anaplastic meningiomas and **papillary meningiomas** are malignant and tend to invade adjacent brain tissue. Symptoms frequently include muscle weakness and other neurological deficits. The incidence of malignant meningiomas is very low. They usually arise over the convexity or in the parasagittal region. Generally, radiation therapy is given in addition to surgery, either alone or with chemotherapy in clinical trials.

Metastatic Brain Tumor
(Separate publication available. See page 137)

A metastatic (secondary) brain tumor is formed by cancer cells that began elsewhere in the body and traveled to the brain. Cancers that frequently spread to the brain include:

▸ lung cancer
▸ breast cancer
▸ colon cancer
▸ melanoma
▸ kidney cancer

A metastatic brain tumor can appear anywhere in the brain or spine. Multiple tumors are common.

If the primary cancer is under control, surgery or radiation can be used to treat single brain tumors. Radiation is the standard treatment for multiple tumors. Chemotherapy may also be used in addition to either surgery or radiation therapy.

Neuroblastoma, Cerebral

The neuroblastoma more commonly occurs outside the central nervous system. The intracranial form is a malignant, rapid growing tumor, commonly causing seizures, focal deficits, and increased pressure within the brain. It is common for them to spread throughout the central nervous system via the cerebrospinal fluid.

Eighty-five percent of cerebral neuroblastomas occur in children and 15% occur in adults. In children, the most common location is in the cerebral hemispheres (see the diagram on page 10).

The neuroblastoma may be called a PNET (primitive neuroectodermal tumor) by some. It is diagnosed by CT or MRI scans, which often shows surrounding edema and calcification.

Combination therapy consisting of surgery, radiation therapy and chemotherapy may be required. If metastases are present, treatment to the entire brain and spine is performed.

Neurocytoma, Central

This rare, grade I, benign tumor typically occurs in a lateral ventricle in the region of the foramen of Monro, and occasionally extends into the third ventricle as well. It is supplied by many blood vessels. The central neurocytoma shows mature cells, similar to normal neurons of the gray matter, although their cell of origin is unknown. It is most common in young adult males. Symptoms are those associated with increased intracranial pressure: headache, nausea and vomiting, drowsiness, vision problems and mental changes.

Standard treatment is surgery, which is often successful. Excessive bleeding can limit the extent of tumor removal however. The routine use of radiation therapy as an adjuvant therapy is still under discussion.

Neurofibromatosis (NF)

The term neurofibromatosis refers to two different genetic diseases. Neurofibromatosis type I, also called NF-1 or von Recklinghausen's Disease, is the more common of the two disorders. It causes tumors called *neurofibromas* to form on nerves throughout the body, and skin discolorations called *café-au-lait* spots. **Optic gliomas** are associated with NF-1.

NF-2 causes tumors to form in the central nervous system, particularly **bilateral acoustic neuromas** (tumors of the 8th cranial nerve). **Meningiomas**, **ependymomas** and tumors of other cranial nerves may also develop. NF-2 may be inherited or may arise independently.

Patients with bilateral 8th nerve tumors, or a single acoustic neuroma, an optic glioma, or a meningioma, are examined to determine if they have NF.

For more information, contact the National Neurofibromatosis Foundation ▾ 95 Pine Street, 16th Floor ▾ New York, NY 10005 ▾ (800) 323-7938 ▾ E-mail nnff@nf.org ▾ http://www.nf.org *or* Neurofibromatosis, Inc. ▾ 8855 Annapolis Road, Suite 110 ▾ Lanham, MD 20705 ▾ (800) 942-6825 ▾ E-mail nfinc1@aol.com ▾ http://www.nfinc.org

Oligodendroglioma

(Separate publication available. See page 137)

These tumors arise from oligodendrocytes, a type of supportive brain tissue. They most frequently occur in young and middle-aged adults but are also found in children. They are slightly more common in men than women. The most common site is one of the cerebral lobes (50% occur in the frontal lobe) and seizures are the most common initial symptoms. This tumor represents about 4% of all primary brain tumors.

Pure oligodendrogliomas are rare. **Mixed gliomas**, tumors containing both oligodendrocytes and astrocytes, are far more common. Oligodendrogliomas often contain a large amount of mineral deposits, called calcification.

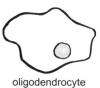
oligodendrocyte

The cells of the well-differentiated oligodendroglioma look only slightly abnormal when viewed under a microscope. It tends to be a slow growing tumor. An **anaplastic (malignant) oligodendroglioma** has very abnormal looking cells, and is faster growing. In rare instances, glioblastoma multiforme cells are found in these tumors.

Oligodendrogliomas might be graded on a scale of A through D or I through IV, depending on the classification system used. The grade represents the most malignant type of cell found in the tumor.

Standard treatment for accessible tumors is surgical removal of as much tumor as possible. Biopsy alone will be done to confirm the specific tumor type with inaccessible tumors. Radiation therapy might follow. Combination chemotherapy using PCV *(procarbazine, CCNU* and *vincristine)* can be beneficial against anaplastic oligodendroglioma. Clinical trials are available using various chemotherapies and radiation therapy. Recurrent tumors can be treated with a second surgery, radiation therapy, chemotherapy or biologic therapy.

Pineal Region Tumors

The pineal gland is located at the rear of the third ventricle. Pineal region tumors represent fewer than 1% of all primary brain tumors. However, 3% to 8% of childhood brain tumors occur in this area.

Tumors occurring in this location include **germinomas**, **teratomas** and other **germ cell tumors**, **astrocytomas**, and **pineal tumors**. See also the listings for individual tumor types.

Pineal Tumors

▲ Pineocytoma
▲ Pineoblastoma
▲ Mixed Pineal Tumor

The **pineocytoma** is a slow-growing, grade II tumor. **Pineoblastoma** is the malignant, grade IV form of this tumor.

Symptoms are most often due to obstruction of cerebrospinal fluid flow causing increased pressure in the brain, and involvement of the optic pathways. Headache, nausea and vomiting, listlessness and double vision are common.

Surgery is possible in some individuals. If not, biopsy alone for diagnosis is performed. The standard treatment for these tumors is radiation therapy. Either conventional radiation or radiosurgery might be used. Chemotherapy plus radiation is often recommended for a pineoblastoma. If hydrocephalus is present, steroids are also prescribed. A shunt procedure might be necessary if the hydrocephalus is not controlled by steroids. Clinical trials are available.

Pituitary Tumors

(Separate publication available. See page 137)

Pituitary adenomas are benign, slow growing tumors of the pituitary gland. They represent about 15% of all primary brain tumors. Pituitary adenomas occur at any age but are rare before puberty. Most of these tumors grow in the front two-thirds of the pituitary, called the adenohypophysis. They often invade the optic chiasm. The most common symptoms of optic chiasm involvement are visual loss and headaches.

Pituitary adenomas are classified as secreting or non-secreting. The majority are secreting tumors and are further classified by the hormone secreted. Because hormones affect other parts of the body, treating a pituitary tumor is a team effort involving many medical specialists.

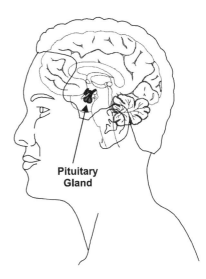

Pituitary Gland

For a prolactin-secreting pituitary adenoma, the drug bromocriptine might be used to reduce the tumor's size. Other drugs to shrink the tumor might be administered depending on the type of hormone the tumor is secreting. Complete surgical removal is the standard treatment for a tumor not controlled by drug therapy. Radiation therapy, following partial surgical removal, or instead of surgery, might be recommended. Radiosurgery is also used. Replacement hormone therapy is often prescribed following surgery and/or radiation. This treatment is usually managed by an endocrinologist, a physician specializing in the hormone balance of the body.

The **pituitary carcinoma** is the rare malignant form of the pituitary adenoma. It is diagnosed only when there are proven metastases. Symptoms are identical to those of the adenoma, and this tumor might also secrete a variety of hormones. Treatment might include surgery, radiation therapy, hormone therapy and chemotherapy.

PNET
Primitive Neuroectodermal Tumor

PNET is a name used for tumors which appear identical under the microscope to the medulloblastoma, but occur primarily in the cerebrum. PNET is used by some to designate tumors such as the **pineoblastoma, polar spongioblastoma,**

medulloblastoma and **medulloepithelioma**. With the exception of the medulloblastoma, all of these are very rare tumors.

PNETs most frequently occur in very young children. The tumors contain undeveloped brain cells, are highly malignant, and tend to spread throughout the central nervous system.

PNETs commonly contain areas of dead tumor cells (necrosis) and cysts. Laboratory tests help differentiate this tumor from other types. CT scans can show cysts and areas of calcification which are common in PNETs. Surrounding edema is uncommon. MRI scans can provide an indication of tumor size.

Because they tend to be large tumors, symptoms of increased intracranial pressure and mass effect are usual. Seizures are common.

Surgery is the standard initial treatment for these tumors. Because of their large size and tendency to spread, as well as their extensive blood supply, total surgical removal is rarely achieved. In children older than three and in young adults, radiation therapy routinely follows surgery, with delivery to the entire brain and spine. Doses are similar to those used for medulloblastoma. Younger children are often treated with chemotherapy instead of radiation therapy, until they are older.

The chemotherapy used for medulloblastoma might also be effective against a PNET. Many clinical trials using chemotherapy and combinations of therapy are available for the medulloblastoma and PNET.

Pseudotumor Cerebri
(Benign intracranial hypertension)

The cause of this condition is unknown, but it is not due to a brain tumor. Pseudotumor cerebri literally means "false brain tumor"—it is increased pressure within the brain. It is most common in women between the ages of 20 and 50.

Headaches, vision changes and other symptoms of increased intracranial pressure are present. Researchers are studying the relationship between obesity, hormone imbalances, ventricular malformations, abnormal vitamin A levels, and/or family histories of this disease to learn more about the origins of this disorder.

Diagnosis is usually confirmed by spinal tap. Scans are used to rule out an actual tumor. Treatment consists of relieving the symptoms. Pressure can be controlled by repeated spinal taps to remove excess fluid, or a shunt. Steroids can be used to reduce swelling of brain tissue. Hyperosmotic drugs (drugs which cause fluids to drain out of body tissue) are used to reduce fluid build-up.

Both the onset and disappearance of symptoms may be spontaneous.

For more information, contact the Pseudotumor Cerebri Society ▾ 750 E. Adams Street ▾ Syracuse, NY 13210 ▾ (315) 464-3937 ▾ http://members.aol.com/ptcsociety/homepage/

Recurrent Tumors

Many malignant tumors cannot be removed completely during surgery because they have spread into surrounding tissues. If they recur, a second surgery may be recommended. Conventional radiation therapy can be given if it was not used as an initial treatment. A form of local radiation therapy, such as implants or radiosurgery might be recommended if conventional radiation therapy has already been given. Chemotherapy is also used to treat recurrent tumors. Clinical trials with chemotherapy, biologic response therapy, and gene therapy are available.

Almost any brain or spinal tumor might recur, although for some types recurrence is very rare. Recurrence rates vary with the type of tumor, its location and the extent of the surgical resection. It is possible for a lower grade tumor to recur as a higher grade especially in astrocytomas, oligodendrogliomas and meningiomas.

In general, treatment for recurrent tumors includes some combination of:

- » surgery
- » standard radiation therapy if not previously received
- » other radiation therapy techniques such as interstitial radiation, radiosurgery or stereotactic radiotherapy
- » chemotherapy
- » biologic therapies
- » gene therapies

Many clinical trials are investigating treatments for recurrent tumors.

Skull Base Tumors

Tumors located along the bones that form the bottom of the skull, or along the bony ridge in back of the eyes are called skull base tumors. These tumors are most often **chordomas, meningiomas, glomus jugulare, schwannomas** or

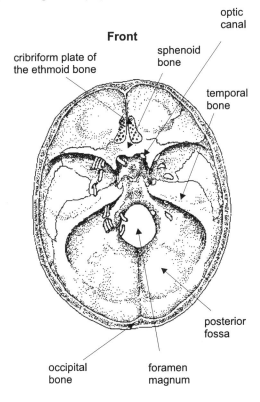

Skull Base

metastatic tumors.

Skull base tumors are diagnosed by scan images. Treatment depends on the type and loca-

tion of the tumor, and its surgical accessibility. Newer surgical tools and stereotactic techniques help the neurosurgeon remove large portions of the tumor. A team approach might be used with extensive tumors: a neurosurgeon, an ear, nose and throat (otorhinolaryngology) specialist, a surgeon with training in cranio-facial surgery, and/or a plastic surgeon.

Outcome depends on the extent of tumor removal and the type of tumor. Recurrent tumors might be treated with a second surgery or focused radiation. Radiation might also be used for partially removed or metastatic tumors.

Spinal Cord Tumors

The types of tumors found in the spine vary by location. Common tumor types include **metastatic tumors, chordomas, schwannomas, meningiomas, astrocytomas** and **ependymomas**.

Primary spinal cord tumors are most often intradural and extramedullary (between the meninges and the surface of the spinal cord).

Some symptoms of spinal tumors are due to compression of the spinal cord and usually have a gradual onset. Muscle weakness is common. If the tumor infiltrates the spinal cord, pain is common.

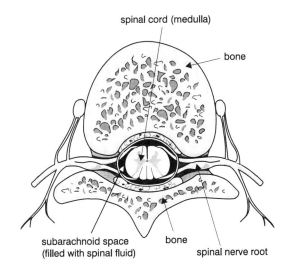

Cross Section of Vertebra and Spinal Cord

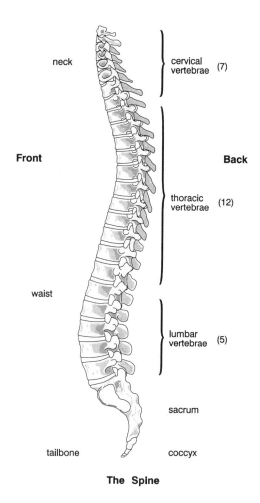

neck

cervical vertebrae (7)

Front

Back

thoracic vertebrae (12)

waist

lumbar vertebrae (5)

sacrum

tailbone

coccyx

The Spine

Treatment of spinal tumors depends on whether the tumor is primary or metastatic, its exact location and type. Surgery is the standard treatment for intradural, extramedullary tumors arising in the spinal canal. Malignant, partially resected, metastatic or inoperable tumors are usually treated with radiation therapy. Chemotherapy might also be used.

Teratoma (Mature)

The mature teratoma is a rare, benign **germ cell tumor** which most frequently occurs in male infants and children. It is the most common brain tumor in newborns. The majority of teratomas occur in children younger than nine, but 20% occur in those between 16 and 18, and almost all occur before age 36. Teratomas represent 18-20%

of all germ cell tumors. A teratoma often contains calcification and cysts. Its most frequent locations are near the third ventricle in the midline—the pineal and suprasellar regions. Germ cell tumors tend to spread via the cerebrospinal fluid. MRI scans with gadolinium contrast and evaluation of the cerebrospinal fluid for tumor cells help determine if the tumor has spread.

Suprasellar tumors often produce symptoms that include diabetes insipidus, vision changes and endocrine dysfunction. Pineal area tumors cause headache, and symptoms of increased intracranial pressure.

Because hydrocephalus occurs in most patients with pineal region tumors, a shunt is often needed to reduce the size of the ventricles before any other treatment can be performed. Surgery is the standard treatment for accessible tumors and can be curative. If surgery is not practical, a biopsy to establish an exact diagnosis might be possible. Radiation therapy may follow surgery or be used for inoperable or partially removed tumors. For children under the age of three, chemotherapy to delay radiation might be recommended.

Toxoplasmosis

This is a generalized infection of the central nervous system caused by a small parasite, Toxoplasma gondi. The parasite is found in the intestines of cats and in uncooked meats. Most people can be exposed to this parasite and never develop symptoms. At risk for severe disease are individuals with compromised immune systems such as AIDS patients, those who have undergone organ transplants, and those who, for other reasons, have a weakened immune system.

The disease is usually diagnosed by a blood test (IgM-IFA) and CT or MRI scan.

Treatment consists of drugs aimed at controlling the infection, including sulfa and anti-parasitic agents. Drug treatment may continue indefinitely in AIDS patients because of the likelihood of recurrence. Blood tests are used to monitor drug levels. Steroids can be given to control swelling of brain tissue.

Tuberous Sclerosis
(Bourneville's Disease)

This is a hereditary, autosomal dominant disorder. This means that a child has a fifty-fifty chance of inheriting tuberous sclerosis if a parent has this disorder. In addition, this disease is the result of a sporadic mutation (the first case in a family) in 50-60% of patients. Tuberous sclerosis becomes obvious in childhood when seizures, skin nodules of the face, and mental retardation become apparent.

Subependymal giant cell astrocytoma is the brain tumor associated with tuberous sclerosis. It often occurs near the foramen of Monro (the narrow channel, also called the interventricular foramen, between the lateral ventricles and the third ventricle through which cerebrospinal fluid flows), and in the head of the caudate. This tumor occurs in 5-7% of patients with tuberous sclerosis. Treatment for this tumor is described in the section on grade I astrocytomas.

Continuing follow-up for tuberous sclerosis and genetic screening for family members is available through tuberous sclerosis clinics.

For additional information, contact the National Tuberous Sclerosis Association ▼ 8181 Professional Place, Suite 110 ▼ Landover, MD 20785 ▼ (800) 225-6872 ▼E-mail ntsa@ntsa.org ▼ http://www.ntsa.org

Uncommon Brain Tumors

With fewer than 35,000 people diagnosed each year in the United States, all *primary* brain tumors are "uncommon." But, some tumors are more rare than others because of their tissue type, or because the tumor developed at an unusual age, or because the tumor grew in an uncommon location.

- Gliomas, tumors that arise from connective tissue of the brain, are the most common primary brain tumors. Astrocytomas, glioblastomas, oligodendrogliomas and ependymomas are all gliomas. Collectively, they account for about 50% of all primary tumors. However, within that large category, choroid plexus tumors and mixed neuronal-glial tumors and several others are uncommon.

- Meningiomas comprise 25%, pituitary tumors 10%, and acoustic neuromas 7.5 %. All other tumor types—chondrosarcoma, chordoma, germinoma, hemangioma, teratoma and others—make up the remaining 7.5%.

- The majority of brain tumors occur in the upper part of the brain, primarily in the cerebral hemispheres. Infratentorial tumors and tumors of the pineal region and ventricles occur less frequently (see diagram on page 12).

- Some brain tumors are more common in children than in adults. When those tumors occur in adults they are considered uncommon. For example, pineal region tumors, medulloblastomas, ependymomas and pilocytic astrocytomas are less common in adults.

Brain tumors are designated an **orphan disease**—a disease with fewer than 200,000 new cases diagnosed in the United States per year.

Chapter 8

Treatment

Your doctor will recommend one or more types of treatment based on the kind of tumor you have, its size and location, your medical history, your age and your overall health.

You or your doctor might want to consult with other specialists before deciding on your treatment plan. If you need help finding a doctor for a second opinion or to inquire about an investigative treatment, call our office at (800) 886-2282 for a Physician Resource List.

This chapter is divided into four sections:

SURGERY
RADIATION THERAPY
CHEMOTHERAPY
BIOLOGIC THERAPIES

SURGERY

▲ What is it and why is it used?

Surgery is the primary treatment for accessible brain tumors (tumors that can be approached without causing severe damage). With this form of treatment, a neurosurgeon removes as much of the tumor as possible.

The purposes of surgery are:
- to cure, whenever possible
- to remove as much tumor as possible
  Even partial removal of a tumor can relieve symptoms, improve quality of life, and decrease the amount of tumor that must be treated by other methods.
- to establish an exact diagnosis
  Tumor cells are examined under a microscope by a pathologist.

- to provide access for other treatments
  Chemotherapy or radiation implants or genetic materials can be inserted into the tumor bed (the site of the removed tumor). Hyperthermia (heat) treatments can be delivered. Preparation for BNCT (boron neutron capture therapy) can be provided.

The goal of surgery is to remove all visible tumor. Many benign tumors are treated only by surgery. Most malignant tumors require additional treatment.

▲ Why wouldn't it be used?

Your doctors consider several factors before deciding whether or not to recommend surgery.
- The location of your tumor: If the tumor is considered to be accessible, it can probably be removed without causing severe neurological damage. Tumors deep in the brain, surrounded by critical structures, or in areas that control language or movement, might be inaccessible.

- The size of the tumor. The number of tumors.
- The tumor's characteristics: Does it have a distinct border or is it spreading?
- Your general health: Can you endure the strain of surgery and anesthesiology? Are your heart, lungs, kidneys and liver functioning well?
- Your neurological status: Do you have signs of increased intracranial pressure?
- If a second surgery is being considered, how long has it been since the first operation?

▲ Before the surgery

The location of your tumor in relation to other structures and blood vessels must be determined as

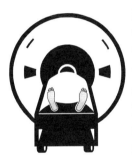

precisely as possible. To achieve this, your doctor will ask you to undergo a variety of tests, which might include CT, MRI or PET scans, and possibly angiography. Using this information, the surgeon can rehearse the operation and plan the safest methods.

▲ Types of surgery

BIOPSY

Biopsy is a surgical procedure to remove a small piece of tumor in order to make a diagnosis. The sample is examined by a pathologist who determines the type of the tumor. A biopsy can be performed as part of the surgery to remove the tumor, or as a separate procedure.

- An **open** biopsy is performed by removing a small portion of the tumor which has been exposed during surgery.
- A **needle biopsy** is performed by making an incision in the skin and then drilling a small hole into the skull. A narrow, hollow needle is inserted through the hole and into the tumor, and a small amount of tumor is drawn up into the needle.

- A **stereotactic needle biopsy** is a needle biopsy accomplished with stereotactic guidance systems—a combination of computers and MRI or CT scanning equipment. The patient's head is placed in a frame which helps direct the path of the needle into the tumor. This type of biopsy is useful for patients with deep or multiple tumors.

CRANIOTOMY

The most commonly performed surgery for removal of a brain tumor is called a craniotomy. "Crani" means skull, "otomy" means cutting into. A portion of the scalp is usually shaved, and an incision is made through the skin. Using high speed drills and a special saw, a piece of bone is removed to expose the area of brain over the tumor. The dura mater (the outermost layer of the meninges) is opened, the tumor is located and then resected (removed). After the tumor is removed, the bone is usually replaced and the scalp stitched shut.

In a **conventional craniotomy**, surgeons guide themselves by what they see, their knowledge of anatomy and their interpretation of the pre-operative scans. In a **stereotactic craniotomy**, computers assist the surgeon.

SHUNT

Some patients with brain tumors develop increased intracranial pressure (IICP). *IICP is discussed in chapter 5, pages 24-25.* To relieve the pressure, a shunt procedure to drain excess or blocked fluid might be required.

A shunt is a narrow piece of flexible tubing (called a catheter) which is inserted into a ventricle in the brain. The other end of the tubing is threaded under the scalp toward the neck, then, still under the skin, threaded to another body cavity where the fluid is drained and absorbed. The body cavities used for drainage are the right atrium of the heart and, more commonly, the abdominal cavity.

A shunt system includes:

▸ a ventricular catheter, which can be detected by x-ray;

▸ an optional reservoir, which allows access to the cerebrospinal fluid (CSF), and can be used to test the shunt device;

▸ a longer catheter, leading to the drainage area; and

▸ a valve system, which permits CSF flow in a single direction only (away from the brain).

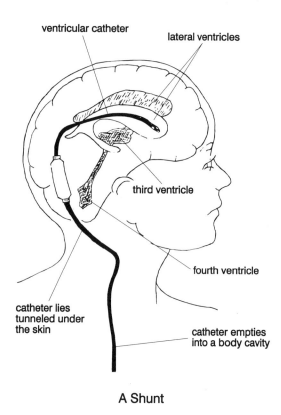

A Shunt

When compared to other brain tumor surgery, the surgery to implant a shunt is relatively minor. A small hole is drilled in the skull through which the catheter is threaded into a ventricle. The shunt valve is tested and then inserted under the scalp. A small incision is made in the abdomen or the chest, depending on which cavity is used for drainage. The other end of the catheter is threaded under the skin to the cavity and then fastened.

Shunts might be temporary—left in place until the brain tumor is surgically removed; or they may be permanent. Shunts are often left in place even after successful surgery.

Following shunt insertion many patients, particularly children, show dramatic improvement within days. In others, symptoms might remain for a period of several weeks.

Each patient receives a set of guidelines describing the signs of shunt malfunction. Your doctor should be notified immediately if any of those signs occur. It might be necessary to correct the problem by a surgical procedure called a shunt revision.

Perhaps only part of the shunt needs correction, such as lengthening the tubing for a growing child. Shunts will require revision or replacement if they are blocked, disconnected, displaced, or if they become infected and do not respond to antibiotic treatment. The need for a shunt revision is not uncommon.

▲ Surgical techniques and tools

A neurosurgeon at a medical center that treats a significant number of brain tumor patients has a wide choice of surgical tools. The most common tools are the surgical laser, ultrasonic aspirator, and operating microscope. Other tools include intraoperative monitoring devices and stereotactic apparatus. The choice of tools depends on the type of tumor and its location, and the surgeon's preference.

BRAIN MAPPING
(Intraoperative monitoring devices)

The scans taken before surgery yield a great deal of information, but they don't always provide the precision needed to avoid critical areas of the brain during the operation. Mapping tools can improve the safety and effectiveness of surgery by locating the exact areas of the brain responsible for speech, comprehension, sensation or movement. Brain mapping is also used to help identify the margin of the tumor and to differentiate between tumor, edema and normal tissue. Brain mapping tools include *direct cortical stimulation, evoked potentials, functional MRI* and *intra-operative ultrasound imaging.*

» **Direct Cortical Stimulation and Somatosensory Evoked Potentials (SSEP)**

In **direct cortical stimulation**, a probe passes a tiny electrical current to delicately stimulate a specific area of the brain, causing a visible movement of the corresponding body part.

Somatosensory-evoked potentials measure the electrical response (evoked potential) of the area. By pre-determining the function of critical areas of brain tissue, those areas can be avoided during surgery and more extensive tumor removal can be achieved.

» **Functional MRI**

This type of MRI (also called Fast MRI) can be an alternative to direct cortical stimulation. The high speed imaging device permits images of the tumor's use of oxygen to be displayed. This helps distinguish between active normal brain and nonactive tumor or necrosis.

» **Intraoperative Ultrasound Imaging**

This technique uses ultrasonic waves during surgery to determine the depth of the tumor and its diameter. It works by sending ultrasound pulses into the brain which then reflect back to the device. The amount of time it takes for the "echoes" to return is measured by a computer and displayed as a TV image. Surgeons can monitor their movements to verify positioning and results during surgery. The waves can also reflect motion such as blood flow.

Ultrasound can make it easier for the surgeon to locate the margins of the tumor so that more extensive tumor removal can be achieved. It helps distinguish between tumor, necrosis (dead tumor cells), cysts, edema and normal brain. Because ultrasound does not readily penetrate bone, it cannot be used pre-operatively.

EMBOLIZATION

Used to reduce the amount of blood supply to a tumor, embolization involves blocking the flow of blood in selected arteries. Arteriography results help determine the need for pre-operative embolization. Surgery follows as soon as possible to avoid re-growth of blood vessels. This technique might be used with vascular tumors such as meningiomas, meningeal hemangiopericytomas and glomus jugulare tumors.

ENDOSCOPY

Endoscopes are long, narrow, flexible tubes. They provide the surgeon with light and visual access as the tube is inserted and directed to the target area.

Pre-operative scans help localize tumors and enable the surgeon to plan surgery using relatively small openings. These small openings (sometimes called keyhole approaches) make it difficult for the surgeon to see. The endoscope helps solve that problem. The neuro-endoscope permits "real-time" visualization, and can also be attached to a surgical laser.

The neuro-endoscope is particularly useful for surgery involving a ventricle—correcting a malfunctioning shunt, removing scar tissue blocking a shunt, or intraventricular tumors. It is also useful during cyst removal.

LASERS

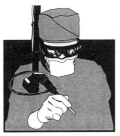

The use of a laser during surgery is relatively routine. This surgical tool aims laser beams at a target and destroys it with heat. Because the light beams cannot penetrate bone, the laser can be used only during surgery.

Lasers are used in addition to, or in place of, a scalpel. Lasers are capable of immense heat and power when focused at close range. Lasers destroy tumor cells by vaporizing them. They are frequently used with stereotactic localization to direct their beams.

The laser's chief uses are with tumors invading the skull base or deep within the brain, with hard tumors which cannot be removed by suction, or with tumors which cannot withstand pulling—tumors that break apart easily. The laser is also used in photodynamic therapy.

MICROSURGERY

Microsurgery is the use of a high-powered microscope during surgery. The surgeon obtains a magnified view of the surgical field. Microsurgery is widely used for brain tumor surgery.

PHOTODYNAMIC THERAPY

Photodynamic therapy combines the use of a sensitizing drug and laser surgery. Prior to surgery, the photosensitizing drug is injected into a vein or artery. It travels through the blood system to the tumor, accumulating in the cells of the tumor. The patient is then taken to surgery for removal of the tumor. During the operation, the treated tumor cells appear fluorescent. The physician aims a laser at the tumor cells, activating the drug. The activated drug then kills the tumor cells.

Only operable tumors can be treated with this procedure. Tumor cells not seen by the surgeon or not sensitive to the drug are not affected by this treatment.

This is a local form of therapy because some parts of the tumor might not be exposed to the light. Because of the danger of swelling, tumors near the brain stem cannot be treated with this technique.

POLYMER WAFER IMPLANTS

To bypass the problem of the blood brain barrier, bio-degradable wafers soaked with a chemo-therapy drug can be used. First, the tumor is re-moved and then wafers are placed into the cavity left by the tumor's removal. The size of the cavity determines the number of wafers used. The surgery is completed as it would be with any other neurosurgical procedure, but the wafers remain in place. The wafers dissolve over time, slowly releasing the chemotherapy directly into the tumor area.

Currently, the drug BCNU is used in these wafers. Future research results might lead to other chemotherapy drugs, anti-angiogenesis drugs (they control the growth of new blood vessels around the tumor), or natural substances such as Taxol to be incorporated into these wafers.

STEREOTACTIC SURGERY

The use of computers to create a three-dimensional image is called **stereotaxy**. Its purpose is to provide precise information about a tumor's location and its position relative to the many structures in the brain. Stereotaxy can be used by the surgeon to map out the surgical procedure beforehand and "rehearse," or by the radiation specialist to plan radiation therapy.

While conventional x-ray pictures depict tumors in two dimensions, stereotaxy provides the third dimension, depth, by obtaining readings in both left to right (coronal) and front to rear (sagittal) directions, then using a computer to analyze the information. It is the third dimension that accurately allows the surgeon to insert the needle for biopsy, the laser beam for vaporization, the scalpel for cutting or the suction device for aspiration.

In the case of biopsy and aspiration, stereo-tactic surgery requires only a small hole (a burr hole) in the skull bone rather than an incision into the brain itself.

Used during surgery, this technique is called **stereotactic surgery**.

Stereotactic surgical techniques are used to biopsy tumors, remove tumors, implant radiation pellets or other local treatments, or to provide a navigational system during surgery (frameless stereotaxy). These techniques are particularly useful in reaching a tumor located deep within brain areas traditionally considered to be difficult to reach, such as the brain stem or thalamus. Stereotaxy can also help limit the extent of surgery by localizing the tumor. Some stereotactic systems can project images of the surgery as it is being performed (**"real time" imaging**).

———

Stereotaxy is performed either with or without a head frame.

» **Head frame**

The technique involves placing the patient's head in a rigid frame so the attached scanning devices can accurately pinpoint the tumor location in three-dimensional space. The rigid frame holds the patient's head in place during the pre-surgical scans and the surgery itself. The information from the CT and/or MRI scans, along with coordinate information from the headframe, is entered into a computer system. The images produced, with their relational coordinates, are used to plan the surgery and guide the surgeon's tools during the procedure.

» **Frameless Stereotaxy**

Frameless navigational systems eliminate the necessity of a headframe. The surgeon touches the brain with a hand-held device during surgery. The device superimposes its location on a computer monitor showing a recent scan or three-dimensional image of the brain. This tool is used to orient the surgeon as to the exact location of the tumor as compared to a specific point on the exterior of the brain.

Viewing Wand

The viewing wand is a computerized, frameless, CT-stereotactic guidance system. It operates in "real-time" by providing location information during surgery continuously and quickly. The surgeon touches a structure in the patient's brain with the wand and a computer program determines the location of relevant areas and displays them on a screen.

This tool is particularly useful during skull base surgery, which is an especially complicated area. It is also of value when multiple tumors are to be removed. The viewing wand can shorten the surgical time by quickly identifying parts of the brain and localizing the tumor.

Compass System (robotic device)

This is a frameless stereotactic system that combines the microscope, laser and computer. The device encircles the patient's head while CT, MRI and angiographic images are obtained. A 3-D map is then created. During surgery, the head holder is placed exactly as it was during the pre-operative studies.

TRANSSPHENOIDAL SURGERY

This type of surgical approach is often used for pituitary adenomas and craniopharyngiomas. *Transsphenoidal means through the sphenoid bone— the skull bone under the eyes and over the nose.* Prior to surgery, the patient undergoes a complete endocrine evaluation. Hormonal disturbances can affect both surgery and recuperation and must be corrected before the operation and monitored afterwards. Incisions under the top lip and through the nasal passage provide access to the sellar area where the tumor is located.

ULTRASONIC ASPIRATION

This tool is used to break tumors apart and then aspirate (suction out) the pieces. Ultrasonic waves cause vibration which fragments the tumor. It causes less disturbance to adjacent tissue than other types of suction devices because it causes less heat and "pull" on normal tissue. This is particularly helpful with tumors that would be difficult to remove with cautery and suction because of their firmness and location. As with the laser, the use of ultrasound has permitted the removal of tumors which would otherwise have been inoperable.

RADIATION THERAPY

▲ What is it and why is it used?

Radiation therapy is a common treatment for brain tumors. It affects both normal and tumor cells, but normal cells are more capable of repairing themselves. As the therapy continues, an increasing number of tumor cells die and the tumor eventually shrinks.

Radiation primarily affects DNA, the basic building material of all cells. Damage to DNA interferes with the cell's ability to divide. Over time, radiated tumor cells die while attempting to reproduce.

Radiation therapy is used:

▸ following surgery for a malignant tumor because stray tumor cells often remain

▸ instead of surgery for an inoperable tumor, or for a tumor that is particularly responsive to this form of treatment

▸ following surgery for benign or malignant tumors if they were not completely removed

▸ to relieve symptoms

▸ to prevent a cancer in another part of the body from developing in the brain

Radiation therapy can be given before or after chemotherapy, before or after surgery, or with drugs that make the tumor more sensitive to radiation.

▲ Why wouldn't it be used?

The brains of **young children** are very susceptible to radiation damage. Chemotherapy is often used to delay radiation therapy until their developing brains can better tolerate it.

With **lower-grade** tumors, particularly those that cause no symptoms, your doctor may recommend a "wait and see" or "watchful waiting" course of action, with close monitoring. Radiation therapy can always be used at a later time if further treatment is needed.

Like any organ in the body, normal brain can tolerate only a limited amount of radiation. When that limit is met, radiation treatments must stop. That is why conventional radiation therapy is rarely repeated. Some form of local radiation (which largely spares normal brain) might be used to treat recurrent tumors.

▲ Conventional treatment machines

▸ *Linear accelerators* are electrical devices that create ionizing radiation in the form of x-rays *(photons)*. The higher the voltage of the device, the more penetrating the x-rays produced. The penetration is essential—otherwise the rays could not reach tumors located deep within the brain behind the bones of the skull.

▸ *Cobalt machines* use cobalt isotopes as the radiation source. A nuclear reactor manufactures the isotopes.

Background

The basis of radiation therapy is the *atom*. The atom consists of several structures. Its nucleus commonly contains protons and neutrons; electrons orbit around the nucleus.

The radiation energy used in medicine creates ions by knocking electrons out of atoms. This is called ionizing radiation. *Ionizing radiation* is medically important because it penetrates and interferes with living tissue.

There are different kinds of ionizing radiation:

▸ *Rays*, including x-rays and gamma rays, are one type. Rays move in waves. They are similar to heat and light waves except the energy is much greater. Rays are also called photon radiation. *"Photon"* refers to light energy. A special electrical device makes *x-rays*. Radioactive isotopes give off *gamma rays*.

▸ Ionizing *particles* are fast moving, tiny pieces of matter, such as neutrons, protons or electrons.

External radiation does not make a person radioactive. Once the waves or particles collide with a target (ideally a tumor cell), the energy is lost and is no longer a threat to the patient or anyone else.

▲ Conventional radiation therapy

Conventional radiation therapy consists of external beams of energy aimed at the tumor. The treatment usually begins a week or two after surgery, or as soon as the surgical wound heals. This type of therapy is usually recommended for a large or spreading tumor.

Conventional radiation is given in divided doses, called *fractions*, over a long period of time. The usual fraction of standard, conventional, external radiation for primary brain tumors is 180–200 cGy. It is given over a six-week period, five days a week. The total dose is usually 5400–6000 cGy (for adults). Lesser amounts of radiation are used to treat metastatic brain tumors. Children also receive fewer cGy.

About Your Radiation Treatment

❖ *Before your treatment begins* a specially trained doctor (a radiation oncologist) reviews your medical records to determine the exact location of your tumor and then plans a treatment based on your situation. To avoid radiating as many healthy cells as possible, the x-rays can be beamed from several different directions or might be computer-shaped to the tumor.

The radiation oncologist might need additional scans or x-rays to verify the target area. Those will be done at a special appointment before you begin your treatments. That visit might also include a planning session called a simulation. Marks made on your skin help the technician properly and consistently direct the treatment machine.

❖ *During your treatment* you will be given the beam radiation on an outpatient basis. Unless radiation is to be delivered to the spine, you will not have to change your clothes.

Radiation therapy is painless. You will not feel, see, or hear anything. A few people notice an unusual smell. Each session consists of a few minutes to aim the machine, and then a few minutes more to deliver the rays. You must remain perfectly still during the treatment. Infants and children might need special equipment or medication to help them keep still.

The average radiation therapy schedule consists of five treatments a week, for five or six weeks. However, other treatment schedules are also used. If you are being treated under one of the other schedules, your doctor will explain it to you.

You are **not radioactive** during or after conventional radiation therapy. There is no need to take any special precautions for the safety of others.

❖ *Results of your therapy* might not be obvious for several months or longer. Tumor cells that have been damaged by radiation cannot reproduce normally and gradually die. The brain clears away the dead tumor cells, but this is a lengthy process.

Scans taken immediately following therapy can be confusing because swelling and dead cells often appear larger than the original tumor, and can cause symptoms similar to the tumor. It takes a few months before scans show the full benefit of the radiation.

Measurement of Radiation
Radiation is measured by the amount of energy absorbed by the body. The unit of measurement is the Gray, abbreviated Gy. Other units of measurement are the centiGray (cGy) and the rad. One cGy equals one rad.

The average x-ray used for diagnosis exposes a person to about .0072 cGy. Radiation used to treat brain tumors is about 6000 cGy (6000 rad).

❖ *Side-Effects* of radiation therapy affect each person differently. You might experience few or none of them and be able to continue working and performing your normal activities. Your radiation oncologist can tell you which, if any, side-effects you are apt to experience, based on your individual treatment plan.

▲ Other types of radiation therapy

BORON NEUTRON CAPTURE THERAPY _____

Boron Neutron Capture Therapy (BNCT) combines a special form of non-ionizing radiation with a drug that concentrates in tumor cells. The drug, when activated by the radiation, kills tumor cells.

The radiation consists of thermal or epithermal (slow) neutron beams. The drug is a boron compound. The boron captures the neutrons, becomes unstable and disintegrates. Cell-killing radiation is then emitted. Normal tissue is spared because the drug remains inactive until it combines with the neutrons. The radiation is harmless unless it activates the boron.

Interest in this form of treatment began more than 25 years ago, but it was not possible to administer it until a radiation beam with the right amount of energy to penetrate effectively was developed. Now, research is centered on finding suitable boron compounds (those without harmful side effects and capable of concentrating in tumor cells only). One form of this treatment has been used on a small number of patients in Japan over the past several years.

In the United States, reactors capable of producing slow neutrons are located in New York, Massachusetts, Georgia, Missouri and Idaho. Some of these centers are offering clinical trials. Call our office at (800) 886-2282 for current information on those trials.

CONFORMAL RADIATION _____

Conformal radiation is high or higher-dose external radiation beams "conformed" to match a tumor's shape and delivered in standard fractions. The beams from a linear accelerator (a conven-tional radiation device) are selectively blocked by computer-customized collimators, blocks, wedges, or the Peacock System. The goal of this new method is to deliver a **uniform** amount of radiation to the entire tumor and to minimize the amount of radiation to other areas of the brain. Tumors not eligible for radiosurgery might be treated with conformal radiation.

Treatments are planned using information from CT scans and highly sophisticated computer programs.

FOCAL RADIATION _____

Focal radiation is high dose radiation, usually given in one fraction, and delivered to an area just encompassing the tumor. The benefit of this therapy is that, while the tumor receives a high dose of radiation, normal tissue is mostly unharmed. *Interstitial radiation* (*brachytherapy*) and *radiosurgery* are two types of focal radiation. The major late complication of these therapies, when used to treat malignant tumors, is development of a symptom-causing mass of dead tumor cells. Surgery to remove those dead cells is required by about 3 or 4 patients out of 10. For more information, see *Interstitial radiation* and *Radiosurgery* in this chapter.

HYPERFRACTIONATED RADIATION THERAPY ____

Tests with large amounts of conventionally fractionated radiation (over 6000 cGy) showed that larger amounts were more effective in controlling brain tumors. However, those same tests also showed an unacceptable increase in long-term side effects.

It is known that brain damage is related not only to higher **total dose**, but also to the **size of the fraction** and to the **volume of brain irradiated**. If the size of each fraction is lowered, or the volume of tissue radiated is decreased, an increase in the total dose might not cause excessive damage. An additional rationale for hyperfractionation is that more frequent fractions allow a better chance of catching a tumor cell in a vulnerable part of the cell cycle.

Conventional fractionation is usually defined as one fraction daily of 180 to 200 cGy, five times a week, for six weeks, for a total dose of 5400 to 6000 cGy. *Hyperfractionation*–more fractions of smaller-than-usual daily doses without a change in overall treatment duration—is used to deliver a larger total dosage. Treatment of brain stem gliomas and malignant gliomas are being studied using hyperfractionation.

HYPERTHERMIA

Hyperthermia is heat therapy. While heat is capable of killing both normal and malignant cells, this technique seeks to heat and kill only tumor cells.

Although tumor cells are no more sensitive to heat than normal ones, several features of tumors make them more prone to damage. These features include poor blood flow, hypoxia (decreased oxygen), and acidity. These same features, often found in the core of a tumor, are responsible for resistance to radiation. This suggests that a combination of heat and radiation can be an effective therapy.

The heat must be carefully administered to get results without undue damage. Heat delivery must be uniform throughout the tumor, with no "hot" or "cold" spots. Normal tissue must be avoided.

Several devices are capable of delivering heat; for example, radiofrequency, microwave, ultrasound and electromagnetic techniques have been used. Researchers are working to determine the most effective heat delivery techniques, but further research remains to be done in this area.

INTERSTITIAL RADIATION THERAPY

This form of therapy is also called *brachytherapy*, *intracavitary radiation*, *radiation implants*, *radiation seeding* or *radioactive pellets*. It consists of implanting sources of radiation energy directly into a tumor. Thus, while standard radiation aims rays at the tumor from outside the body, interstitial radiation attacks the tumor from the inside. The advantage to interstitial radiation is that the effect on normal tissue is greatly reduced. For this type of therapy to be effective, the tumor must be quite small (no more than 2 inches or 5 cm in diameter) and surgically accessible. Larger tumors may require surgery to reduce the size of the tumor before the radiation sources are implanted. Interstitial radiation is a **local** therapy. It is not commonly used for widely spread or multiple tumors.

This type of therapy can be used for newly diagnosed or recurrent tumors, as a boost before or following standard external radiation for newly diagnosed or recurrent tumors.

To implant radiation energy in the tumor, catheters (tubes) are placed into the tumor bed using CT and MRI directed stereotactic surgical techniques. The sources of radiation, usually in pellet form, are placed in the catheters. Depending on the isotopes used, the implant is removed either after a few days, after several months or left in place permanently. Steroids are commonly used with this therapy to decrease brain swelling. Different radioactive isotopes are currently being used as implants and others are being developed.

Follow-up surgery to remove dead tumor cells is required by about 30% – 40% of the patients receiving this therapy.

Unlike external radiation, with interstitial radiation the patient **IS** radioactive and precautions are needed until the implant is removed or until a predetermined amount of time has elapsed

In rare instances, interstitial implants might be repeated.

RADIOACTIVE MONOCLONAL ANTIBODIES

An antibody is a substance produced by white blood cells in response to a foreign object (an *antigen*). The human body often considers tumor cells to be foreign objects because they have unique proteins (antigens). Because an antibody binds only to a specific antigen, it can act as a homing device to a tumor cell. Monoclonal antibodies, manufactured in large quantity in the laboratory, can be mated to radioactive isotopes which kill tumor cells.

Work continues to solve the problems of tumor specificity, delivery across the blood brain barrier, and large cell volume.

RADIOSENSITIZERS AND RADIOPROTECTORS

Radiosensitizers are drugs used before or during radiation therapy to make tumor cells more sensitive or vulnerable to radiation therapy. They do not usually kill tumor cells on their own. This class of drugs, to be useful, must concentrate primarily in tumor rather than normal cells. BUdR, IUdR, hyperbaric oxygen and tirapazamine are examples of radiosensitizers.

Radioprotectors, such as DFMO, are drugs used to protect normal brain cells from the effects of radiation therapy. By protecting normal cells, higher—and hopefully more effective—doses of radiation can be given to destroy tumor cells.

Both types of drugs are being tested primarily in adults whose tumors are being treated with conventional radiation therapy. This includes patients with high-grade astrocytomas, glioblastomas and ependymomas.

RADIOSURGERY

Stereotactic radiosurgery is not surgery—it is a special, focal form of radiation. This treatment allows precisely focused, high dose radiation beams to be delivered to a small brain tumor (usually 1½ inches or less in diameter) in a single treatment session.

Because radiosurgery is radiation and not surgery, the tumor can be located in an area of the brain or spinal cord that might be considered inoperable. If the treatment is delivered in multiple sessions, it is called *fractionated*. Using special computer planning, this treatment minimizes the amount of radiation received by normal brain tissue.

Stereotactic radiosurgery is also used:
▸ as a local "boost" following conventional radiation therapy
▸ for a recurrent tumor when the patient has already received the maximum safe dose of conventional radiation therapy

▸ as a substitute for surgery for a benign tumor (such as a pituitary, pineal region or acoustic tumor)
▸ for a metastatic brain tumor

Prior to treatment, the patient is fitted with a headframe. CT and/or MRI scans are done with the headframe in place to obtain information necessary for treatment planning. Once the planning is completed, treatment can begin.

Radiosurgery is used to treat benign and malignant brain tumors. Possible side-effects of radiosurgery include edema (swelling), occasional neurological problems and radiation necrosis (an accumulation of dead cells). A second surgery to remove the build-up of dead tumor cells may be required.

Three types of machines can deliver this special, focal form of radiation: **Gamma Knife**; **Linac** (adapted linear accelerators); and **Cyclotrons** (proton beam radiosurgery).

» **Gamma Knife Radiosurgery**
The Gamma Knife contains 201 radioactive cobalt sources which can all be computer-focused onto a single area. The patient is placed on a couch and then a large helmet is attached to the headframe. Holes in the helmet allow the beams to match the calculated shape of the tumor. The couch is slid into a globe that contains radioactive cobalt.

The most frequent use of the Gamma Knife has been for small, benign tumors, particularly acoustic neuromas, meningiomas and pituitary tumors. For larger tumors, partial surgical removal might be required first.

The Gamma Knife is also used to treat solitary metastases and small malignant tumors with well-defined borders.

» **Linac Radiosurgery**
An adapted linear accelerator delivers a single, high-energy beam that is computer-shaped to the tumor. The patient is positioned on a sliding bed around which the linear accelerator

circles. The linear accelerator directs arcs of radioactive photon beams at the tumor. The pattern of the arc is computer-matched to the tumor's shape. This reduces the dose delivered to surrounding normal tissue.

» **Proton Beam Radiosurgery (Heavy Particle Radiation Therapy)**

A cyclotron is an adapted nuclear reactor that produces charged particle beams of protons. These beams are used for small, deep-seated tumors such as a pituitary tumor.

The patient is positioned on a table with a fitted facemask in place. As the nuclear reactor smashes atoms, the released protons are directed toward the tumor through blocks which have been computer-programmed to match the beams to the shape of the tumor.

Proton beam radiosurgery appears to have a role in the treatment of skull base and unusually shaped brain tumors. Because malignant brain tumors tend to have irregular borders and stray cells, a precisely confined beam might not be appropriate. Studies are currently being planned to use charged particles (protons) for localized boosts to tumor volumes defined on CT and MRI scans, in much the same way as interstitial implants.

For more information about radiosurgery, contact the International Radiosurgery Support Association ▼ 3540 North Progress Avenue, Suite 207 ▼ Harrisburg, PA 17110 ▼ (717) 671-1701 ▼ Fax (717) 671-1703 ▼ E-mail intouch@irsa.org ▼ http://www.irsa.org

▲ Re-irradiation

Radiation kills normal cells as well as tumor cells. Since brain tissue cannot replace itself, the effects of radiation are cumulative. Only so many normal cells can be killed before severe results occur. For this reason, re-treatment with conventional fractionated radiation is not often recommended. However, re-irradiation is possible in selected circumstances. It depends on the location of the

tumor and its relation to critical brain tissue, when the previous radiation was given, the amount of radiation originally given, the type of tumor and the age of the patient.

Metastatic brain tumors may be re-irradiated because the initial treatment usually involves less than the maximally tolerated dose.

Interstitial radiation therapy and stereotactic radiosurgery are used for re-irradiation of selected patients with recurrent malignant gliomas and metastatic brain tumors after previous conventional fractionated external radiation.

CHEMOTHERAPY

▲ What is it and why is it used?

Chemotherapy uses special drugs to kill tumor cells. Chemotherapy can be a primary (first) therapy or an adjuvant (additional) therapy. For example, when chemotherapy is used to delay radiation treatments for young children, chemotherapy is a primary therapy. As an adjuvant therapy, chemotherapy is given prior to or following other treatments. Chemotherapy is also used to treat recurrent tumors.

▲ Why wouldn't it be used?

There are reasons why chemotherapy might *not* be recommended to treat your tumor.

▶ **Not all brain tumors are sensitive to or respond to chemotherapy.** If it is known that your type of tumor does not respond to chemotherapy, or if, for reasons unknown, it comes to resist the drug that is given, other drugs or treatments will be recommended.

▶ **Chemotherapy affects both normal and tumor cells.** The effect on normal cells is the cause of side-effects. Although side-effects vary with each drug, otherwise good general health—such as acceptable heart, lung and kidney function—is necessary to withstand the rigors of treatment.

▲ How chemotherapy is given

Chemotherapy treatment might be given in the hospital, in out-patient facilities, your doctor's office or your home. Nurses trained in the administration of chemotherapeutic drugs give the medication based on your doctor's orders.

Treatment cycles vary with the drug being given. Your cycle might be one day of treatment followed by a few weeks "off" treatment, or a month "on" chemotherapy and a month "off." The schedule might be repeated only once or twice, or it might continue for a year or longer. A chemotherapy schedule is influenced by two factors: The purpose of the drug and the action of the drug.

The **purpose** of the drug determines when treatment begins. For example, radiosensitizers are drugs which make a tumor more sensitive to radiation therapy. They are used only before or during radiation. On the other hand, drugs used to kill tumor cells might be given before, after, during, or instead of other treatments.

The specific **action** of the drug determines how often the drug needs to be repeated. Cell-cycle specific drugs (see box below) might be given once as a large injection, or might be repeated at regular, short intervals. Non cell-cycle specific drugs work during any phase of the cell cycle. Treatment plans might include a combination of cell-cycle specific and non-specific drugs, depending on the type of tumor.

Your doctor will discuss your treatment plan with you and your family. Consider important details such as the time required to travel to your chemotherapy appointments, the daily activities you need to continue while in treatment, and the effect of potential side-effects. Together, you and your family or friends can form a personalized treatment schedule that works best for your life-style.

Most chemotherapy drugs are given by injection. Injection routes include:

- ▸ intra-arterial = into an artery = IA
- ▸ intracavitary/interstitial = within the cavity left by the removed tumor, placed directly into brain tissue
- ▸ intramuscular = into a muscle = IM
- ▸ intrathecal = into the space between the meninges
- ▸ intratumoral = into the tumor
- ▸ intravenous = into a vein = IV
- ▸ intraventricular = into a ventricle
- ▸ epidural = into the lining of the spine
- ▸ into an implanted device = such as an Ommaya Reservoir

How does chemotherapy work?

Chemotherapy drugs act on DNA—the genetic material found within each cell. The drugs alter the ability of tumor cells to copy their DNA and reproduce.

All cells follow a regular pattern of growth called the cell cycle. The cycle consists of five successive steps, or phases. Each cell that completes the cycle reproduces itself as two new cells. The two cells produce four new cells, four cells produce eight cells, and so on.

In order for a cell to produce normal cells, it must complete specific jobs during each phase of the cell cycle. Each cell must make proteins and enzymes needed to fuel its reproductive process, then duplicate and separate its set of chromosomes. A cell that spends too much or too little time in a phase might not successfully complete the job of that phase. For example, a cell might produce too many proteins or not enough enzymes. (Why this happens is still unknown to scientists.) The abnormal cell continues along the cell cycle. Each abnormal cell is capable of producing two new abnormal cells. Those two cells produce four abnormal cells, four produce eight, until there are enough abnormal cells to form a mass or lump—called a tumor. Chemotherapy is effective when it stops abnormal cells from going through the cell cycle.

Actively dividing cells are the most vulnerable to chemotherapy. Most tumor cells and some normal cells fall into that category. The effect of chemotherapy on normal cells causes the unwanted side-effects. Chemotherapy is usually given in cycles, and the cycles are repeated over a specific period of time. The cycle schedule is designed to allow sufficient time for affected normal cells to recover between treatments.

IMPLANTED PUMPS AND CATHETERS _____

When drugs are going to be repeated over a long period of time, a pump or catheter might be implanted under the skin. This provides continuous access to a vein without repeated needle sticks. The patient is given a local anesthetic and then the doctor makes a small incision. The device is placed under the skin and stitched in place. This procedure can be done at the bedside or in out-patient surgery.

There are many implantable devices on the market. Your doctor will choose one based on the drugs to be used and the treatment schedule. Following placement of the pump or catheter, the nurses instruct the patient on how to care for it.

Pumps are also used to control the flow rate of chemotherapy drugs. A pre-determined amount of drug is attached to the pump, a drop-rate is calculated and set on the machine, and the intravenous tubing attached to the patient's catheter. A beeping monitor alerts the nurse and patient to any change in the calculated rate of flow.

_____

At pre-determined times during your chemotherapy treatment, blood tests will be done. Your doctors use these tests to measure the drug's effect on the normal cells of your body. It is not unusual for a patient's blood test results to be slightly abnormal during treatment, but this does not necessarily alter your treatment schedule. How-ever, if you have any indication of an infection, such as a fever, or experience abnormal bleeding, notify your doctor immediately. Treatment might be stopped temporarily, but can resume once your body recovers. Your doctor might also decide to change the dose or type of chemotherapy. Scans will be done at regular intervals to see if the size of your tumor is changing.

▲ Types of chemotherapy
BLOOD BRAIN BARRIER DISRUPTION _____

The blood brain barrier is a filter mechanism that allows only selected substances into the brain. This works to our advantage when harmful substances, such as certain chemicals or bacteria, are prohibited from entering. It works to our disadvantage when substances we want to enter the brain, such as chemotherapy, are kept out.

Blood brain barrier disruption is a technique used to temporarily disrupt the barrier in order to allow chemotherapy to flow from blood vessels into the brain. A drug such as *mannitol* is used to disrupt the barrier. Chemotherapy drugs are then injected into an artery or a vein and travel through the blood to the brain and into the tumor. The disruption also allows high levels of the drug to enter normal brain as well. This might cause a temporary worsening of symptoms and/or seizures. The barrier is restored naturally as the effects of the mannitol wear off. New agents being developed will be more selective in opening the

---

Blood Brain Barrier

Treating brain tumors with chemotherapy is different from treating tumors elsewhere in the body. The brain has a natural defense system not present in other organs of the body. That system, called the blood brain barrier, protects the brain from foreign substances by blocking their passage from the blood. For a drug to be effective in treating brain tumors, a sufficient quantity must either pass through the blood brain barrier or bypass it entirely.

Some drugs do pass through, or permeate, the blood brain barrier. The group of drugs called nitrosoureas (such as BCNU and CCNU) are such drugs. Procarbazine, temozolomide, platinum-based drugs (such as cisplatin, cisplatinum, or carboplatin) and some natural substances (such as taxol) also cross the barrier. And, researchers are studying ways to disrupt or bypass the blood brain barrier.

blood brain barrier and thus cause fewer side-effects. (See *Receptor-Mediated Permeabilizers* in this chapter.)

This technique is used primarily to treat primary central nervous system lymphoma and high-grade astrocytoma tumors.

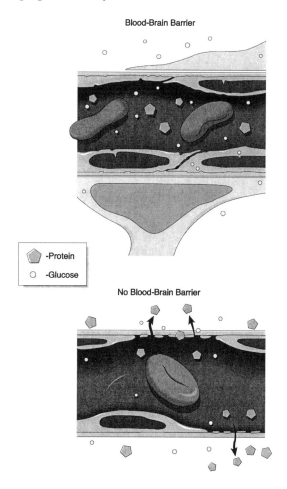

Blood-Brain Barrier

⬠ -Protein
○ -Glucose

No Blood-Brain Barrier

BONE MARROW or STEM CELL TRANSPLANTATION _____

One of the most common side-effects of chemotherapy is damage to the bone marrow—the part of the body that produces new blood cells. The possibility of bone marrow damage influences the amount of drug that can be given.

For patients requiring high-doses of chemotherapy, doctors can transplant healthy bone marrow or stem cells (baby blood cells) after the treatments are completed. This procedure is called a *bone marrow transplant* or *stem cell transplant*. An *autologous* transplant means the patient's own

marrow is used. An *allogenic* transplant uses marrow from a donor. With the patient under anesthesia, the doctor extracts marrow from the pelvic bone using a needle and syringe. This procedure is called harvesting. *Peripheral stem cell rescue* uses stem cells from blood instead of bone marrow cells.

Following the harvesting of the bone marrow or stem cells, an intensive course of high-dose chemotherapy is given over several days. After therapy is complete, the marrow or stem cells are given to the patient through an intravenous solution. The marrow begins producing a new supply of blood cells or the stem cells begin to mature into adult blood cells and reproduce. *Colony stimulating factors* (CSFs) might be used to help control the body's natural tendency to reject the transplanted marrow.

Bone marrow transplantation was developed to treat childhood leukemia; it is now available to adults and children with medulloblastomas or glioblastomas. Due to the complexity of this treatment, transplantation should be done at an experienced institution with a multi-disciplinary team. The team can assist with donor matching, supportive counseling, family member housing during treatment, and financial counseling.

For more information, a patient manual and newsletters are available from the Blood & Marrow Transplant Newsletter ▾ 1985 Spruce Ave ▾ Highland Park, IL 60035 ▾ (847) 831-1913 ▾ Fax (847) 831-1943 ▾ http://www.bmtnews.org Those seeking a bone marrow donor or wishing to donate marrow can register with the National Marrow Donor's Registry at (800) 654-1247.

COMBINATION CHEMOTHERAPY _____

Drugs may be given in combination

▸ to increase effectiveness, especially if the drugs chosen differ in their modes of action and the side-effects they cause

▸ the combination of several drugs might serve to control all the tumor cell types present

▸ two or more drugs in combination might be more effective than when they are used alone

HIGH-DOSE CHEMOTHERAPY

Massive doses of chemotherapy are administered, then an antidote is given which reverses, or "mops up," the excess drug. Methotrexate is the drug most often used for high-dose chemotherapy, and Leucovorin is the most common antidote. This technique is offered to those with high-grade astrocytomas or primary central nervous system lymphomas.

HORMONE THERAPIES

Tamoxifen and *RU-486* are two hormone therapies used to treat brain tumors. They work by inhibiting tumor growth.

- Tamoxifen (Nolvadex or Tamofen) is an anti-estrogen drug that appears to inhibit cell growth. It is being tested in high doses against recurrent malignant gliomas.
- RU-486, also called mifepristone, is an anti-progesterone. It is currently being tested with some meningiomas.

INTRACAVITARY/INTERSTITIAL THERAPY

The administration of chemotherapy directly into a tumor is called intracavitary or interstitial therapy. Among the various methods used are implanted catheters and polymer wafer implants placed during surgery. These techniques have the potential advantage of reducing the amount of drug affecting normal cells in the brain and throughout the body, and increasing the amount of drug reaching tumor cells.

LOWER TOXICITY DRUGS

A new generation of chemotherapy drugs with lower levels of toxicity (side effects) are being explored for malignant brain tumors. Included in that category are the drugs temozolomide and phenylacetate.

MICROSPHERES

Controlled-release drugs offer relief from repeated injections. Researchers are designing a microencapsulation system which will "package" several doses of drug into one capsule. The system might also be capable of "layering" several drugs into one capsule. The capsules, called microspheres, are designed to dissolve slowly and release their contents over a pre-determined amount of time. Not yet available for brain tumor patients, the capsules are designed to be given by injection or orally.

RECEPTOR-MEDIATED PERMEABILIZERS (RMPs)

Receptor-Mediated Permeabilizers (RMPs) offer another way of delivering drugs through the blood brain barrier. RMPs are synthetic substances modeled after naturally occurring compounds. These substances temporarily increase the openings of the blood brain barrier, allowing drugs to pass into the brain. In addition, early studies indicate that RMPs *selectively* permeate the barrier, showing promise of increasing drug delivery to the tumor while reducing side-effects to healthy brain tissue.

The technique involves giving the chemotherapy drug by injection, followed by an injection of the RMP. Studies of one RMP, called RMP-7, are underway in the United States for patients with certain metastatic brain tumors. (See also Blood-Brain-Barrier and Blood-Brain-Barrier Disruption in this chapter.)

RESERVOIRS

Chemotherapy can be delivered directly into the cerebrospinal fluid, bathing the brain and spinal cord with drugs. This treatment is used for meningeal tumors involving the ventricles or spine, or tumors that tend to "seed" down the spine. A small "container" such as an Ommaya Reservoir is surgically placed under the scalp. A tube leads from the reservoir into a ventricle of the brain. Medications are injected via syringe into the reservoir and then the reservoir is pumped. The pumping begins the flow of drug through the ventricles and lining of the spine. Chemotherapy administered this way can be repeated on a regular schedule.

The Immune System

The immune system is composed of several different types of cells.

▸ **Lymphocytes**—the main type of immune cell, are a type of white blood cell. They produce the **interferons**.

   » **B cells**—are lymphocytes that circulate in the blood like soldiers on patrol. When they find an antigen (a stranger presumed to be harmful), they manufacture a specific weapon, called an **antibody**, against it. Antibodies are proteins that recognize and attach to antigens and destroy them.

   » **T cells**—are lymphocytes that directly attack targeted foreign invaders. They also circulate in the blood. T cells direct and regulate the immune response by signaling other immune system defenders. T cells produce proteins called **lymphokines**, which are a type of **cytokine**. Cytokines are chemical substances that control a number of cell activities, including the immune response. The **interleukins** are released from T lymphocytes and macrophages.

   » **NK** (natural killer) cells—destroy cancer cells by producing chemical substances that bind to and kill any foreign invaders. The destroyed tumor cells are absorbed by **phagocyte** cells.

   » **LAK** (lymphokine activated killer cells) are "super charged" natural killer cells created in the laboratory by exposing NK cells to IL-2.

▸ **Monocytes**—are white blood cells that travel into tissues and develop, when needed, into **macrophages**, as part of the immune response. Monocytes and macrophages play a key role in **phagocytosis**, a process by which some cells "eat" other cells and foreign invaders. Macrophages produce **tumor necrosis factor** (TNF) which can kill tumor cells directly or cause damage to blood vessels thereby interfering with the tumor's supply of oxygen and food.

Biological therapies used to treat tumors target some of these defenses—boosting, directing, or restoring the body's own tumor-fighting mechanisms.

Adapted from NCI's Cancer Facts: Biological Therapies and
American Brain Tumor Association: Immunotherapy of Brain Tumors

---

BIOLOGIC THERAPIES

▲ What is it?

Biologic therapy seeks to make it difficult for tumors to grow by changing their biological environment or by changing their behavior. This therapy uses substances called **biological response modifiers** (BRMs). Many BRMs occur naturally in the body. They act in several different ways, including:

▸ enhancing the body's immune system to fight tumor growth

▸ changing cellular signals that permit tumor growth

▸ making tumors more susceptible to destruction by the immune system

▸ reversing or blocking the process that changes normal cells into cancer thereby altering the abnormal growth behavior of a tumor

Biologic therapies are being actively investigated for use against glioblastoma multiforme, malignant astrocytomas and many other types of tumors.

▲ Types of biologic therapies

ANGIOGENESIS INHIBITORS

Once a tumor reaches a certain size, it cannot continue to grow without increased biological supplies such as oxygen and food. At that time, the tumor produces special proteins that promote angiogenesis (the growth of new blood vessels). The new vessels increase the tumor's supply lines, enabling it to continue growing.

Angiogenesis (angio=blood vessel; genesis=birth) inhibitors, also called anti-angio-genesis therapy, block the development of new blood vessels and disrupt the new vessels already formed. Without adequate supply lines, the tumor stops growing.

The following anti-angiogenesis agents are under investigation: **Angiostatin** and **Endostatin**; **Paclitaxel**; **Platelet Factor 4 (PF4)**; **Squalamine**; and **Thalidomide**. Some of these agents are being offered in clinical trials.

ANTI-SENSE THERAPIES

This form of gene therapy seeks to block specific protein messages formed by malignant cells. The targeted messages interrupt normal growth of the cell. If the abnormal messages can be blocked, so can the growth of the tumor. Short fragments of DNA (genetic material), called oligodeoxy-nucleotides, can stop the formation of the harmful messages.

DIFFERENTIATORS

Mature cells are said to be "differentiated." They know their place and function, and perform it. Immature cells are still "growing up" and can be influenced into becoming something they weren't meant to be. Still other cells are "undifferentiated" or "de-differentiated." They have either regressed from a more mature state, or never grew up. Cancer cells are undifferentiated or de-differen-tiated. Agents that seek to make cancer cells more differentiated (or normal) are called differentiating agents.

Examples of this type of drug are the retinoids such as **Accutane** (a derivative of Vitamin A), and **phenylbutyrate/phenylacetate.**

GENE THERAPY

(Separate publication available. See page 137)
Genes, part of the genetic material called DNA, carry the instructions for making proteins involved in cell growth.

Genes sometimes become abnormal and might produce defective proteins that cause tumors. Gene therapy seeks to repair or replace those defective genes. Three methods are currently being tested in patients: the suicide gene, the immune enhancer gene and tumor suppressor genes such as p53.

The **suicide gene**, carried to the tumor by a harmless virus, slightly changes the tumor's genetic structure so that a unique protein is produced. An anti-viral drug is then given which converts the protein into a toxin that kills the tumor cells.

The **immune enhancer gene** is injected into the tumor. It produces an immune response against the tumor.

The **tumor suppressor gene**, carried to the tumor by a virus, can restore normal function to existing but changed tumor suppressor genes or replace missing genes.

GROWTH FACTORS

Growth factors are substances that promote cell growth. Some growth factors are produced by and affect the same tumor cell. Others are produced by a second cell. **Transforming growth factors** and the **interleukins** are both growth factors. Manipu-lating growth factors or their receptors and the effects of doing so is the focus of many research efforts.

IMMUNOTOXIN THERAPY

An immunotoxin is created by linking a poison (toxin) to an antibody or other substance that can carry it directly to the tumor. Research on the transferrin-diptheria toxin and pseudomonas toxin is continuing.

INTERFERONS

Interferons are proteins produced by lymphocytes and occur naturally in the body. The three families of interferons are the alpha, beta and gamma. These biological substances are thought to inhibit tumor cell growth by stimulating the production of B cells. The interferons are also thought to be angiogenesis inhibitors.

Most of the research into the interferons combines them with various chemotherapy drugs.

INTERLEUKINS

The interleukins are proteins produced by T lymphocytes and macrophages. There are many naturally occuring interleukins, including IL-1 through IL-15. Together, they help coordinate the activities of the immune system.

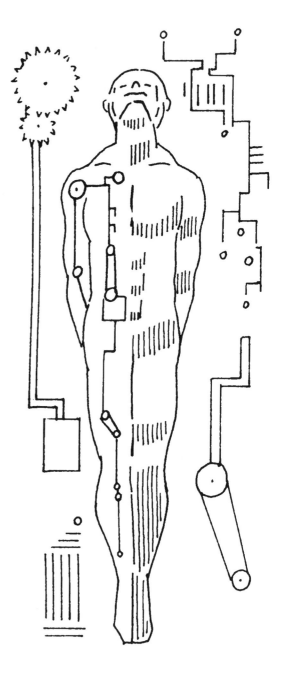

IL-2 stimulates immune cells such as lymphocytes that can destroy tumor cells. IL-2 stimulated lymphocytes are called **LAK** (lymphokine-activated killer cells). Lymphocytes are removed from the patient's blood, stimulated with IL-2 in the laboratory, and then returned to the patient as LAK cells. Clinical studies of the interleukins are ongoing.

Chapter 9

Clinical Trials

In hundreds of laboratories throughout the world, researchers screen countless numbers of plants, biologicals, synthetic substances and high-tech devices looking for new ways to effectively treat brain tumors. When a substance or technique shows promise, it may be developed for testing in patients.

New treatments are tested on patients in *clinical trials*—organized programs designed to determine the safety and effectiveness of a new therapy. The trials might be funded by the National Institutes of Health, pharmaceutical companies, or by a single institution.

Background

Clinical trials might be conducted by a single institution, or by several institutions acting as a single unit—a *clinical cooperative group or consortium.*

Because of the relative rarity of brain tumors, many single institutions could not enter sufficient numbers of patients into a clinical trial to derive meaningful data or would take a long time to do so. Clinical cooperative groups and consortia were created by the National Cancer Institute to overcome these obstacles.

▲ Protocols

All patients enrolled in a clinical trial must meet the same entry criteria, receive the same treatment, and be evaluated the same way. That "sameness" enables researchers to objectively measure the results of a new treatment. A clinical trial uses a pre-defined, written plan of treatment called a *protocol* to help ensure consistency.

A protocol includes:
- ▸ the goals of the study
- ▸ the number of patients that must be enrolled for the study to be meaningful

- ▸ the entry criteria, which specifies:
  - » the types of tumors to be treated
  - » any exclusions due to previous treatments
  - » acceptable age ranges
  - » overall health requirements
- ▸ a detailed explanation of how the treatment is to be given
- ▸ how patient progress is to be evaluated

An appropriate source, such as the National Cancer Institute (NCI) or the Food and Drug Administration (FDA), approves the testing of the new treatment. Because clinical trials are considered experimental even when using or combining older drugs in new ways, the committee that reviews human testing at each participating hospital (the IRB or Institutional Review Board) must also give their approval. Patients who are considering the new treatment must be "informed" and sign an "informed consent" form if they want to participate.

Only specially authorized physicians, called **clinical investigators**, are allowed to administer the new treatment.

Those who enter clinical trials not only help research to advance, but they have the first chance to benefit from improved, state-of-the-art treatment methods.

If a clinical trial shows that its new treatment is better than the standard treatment in use, the new treatment might become the standard treatment.

> ### Informed Consent
> Prior to any kind of treatment, the patient has a *right* to know the exact nature of the treatment, known risks, the prospects of success and if there are alternative methods of treatment. Informed consent means that the information must be **explained** to the patient by a doctor or nurse and the patient must fully **understand** the explanation. Parents or guardians may substitute for minors.

▲ A Note About Entry Criteria

Sometimes a person finds they don't meet the entry criteria and are therefore not "eligible" for a specific clinical trial. This may happen for several reasons.

▸ Because most clinical trials are *treatments*, patients are generally required to have growing tumors. Trials are open to those with newly diagnosed tumors or those whose tumors were treated and are now growing again.

▸ The results of a blood test may have been outside of acceptable range, or the tumor type isn't being treated in the trial.

▸ The trial might have filled quickly and is now closed to new patients.

Learning that you or your loved one cannot be treated in a specific clinical trial can be very upsetting. Everyone wants the newest treatments medicine can offer.

If you are ineligible for the clinical trial you wanted to enter, please remember:

▸ The media often portray new research as a "cure," long before anyone knows whether it is or isn't. If the new treatment was proved to be a "cure," a clinical trial wouldn't be needed. Only clinical trials can furnish that proof.

▸ If one trial has closed, look for another. Entry criteria is different for each clinical trial and

there are over 200 brain tumor trials currently entered in the National Cancer Institute's clinical trials database.

▲ Phases

Clinical trials are conducted in phases. Each phase focuses on answering a specific question about the new treatment.

PHASE I TRIAL

The purpose of a Phase I trial is to find out **how much** of the new substance can be safely given and the best way to give it. A small number of patients (15–25) with various kinds of tumors receive the experimental treatment.

Although the research team monitors the patient carefully, no one knows the effectiveness or risks of the new treatment. Phase I treatments might have anti-tumor effects, although that is not the primary purpose of the phase.

As doctors monitor the effect of the new treatment on the overall health of the patient, treatment dosages might be adjusted. Blood, urine, and other tests outlined in the protocol are performed frequently to monitor for side-effects. As the trial continues, the dosage is slowly increased. When a balance is reached between dosage and side-effects, the treatment moves into a Phase II study.

Phase I/II trials also exist: if the drugs under investigation are well known in other diseases, but the correct dosages with brain tumors have yet to be determined, phases I and II may be combined.

PHASE II TRIAL

The purpose of a Phase II study is to determine **effectiveness**. Phase II studies are offered to patients with very specific types of tumors. Although the majority of patients have already received conventional treatment and now require additional treatment, an increasing number of trials are open to newly diagnosed patients.

The study stays open until the entry of about 20–50 patients with each tumor type to be tested. After the pre-determined number of patients is enrolled, the trial closes. Patients are monitored according to the protocol outline and side-effects are carefully evaluated. An effective treatment is one in which patients' tumors stop growing or shrink in size.

PHASE III TRIAL

If the new treatment is found to be effective and appears to be safe, it moves to Phase III. This phase **compares the new treatment to the standard treatment** to determine which is more effective. A large number of patients are entered into Phase III studies so that the effectiveness of the different treatments, called *treatment arms*, can be statistically measured and compared.

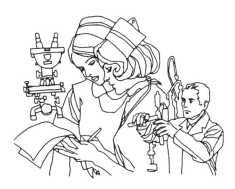

Investigators in a clinical trial share their information throughout the duration of the protocol. The data can be communicated verbally, posted on the Internet, presented at medical conferences, and/or published in medical journals. If the treatment is found to be ineffective or harmful, notice is communicated immediately to all doctors and patients involved. If the treatment seems to be a significant improvement over the standard treatment, that also is immediately shared.

▲ Types of trials

RANDOMIZED STUDY

If the trial is a randomized study, the treatment arm (standard versus new) assigned to each patient is determined by a computer. This random assignment process eliminates bias and ensures that an equal number of patients receive each treatment.

The term "bias" is used here in the statistical sense. The problem is that doctors might select therapies for their patients in a way that tends to invalidate the results of the study. For example, the youngest and healthiest patients might be chosen for the most aggressive and riskiest therapy. Then, if the therapy looks promising, it might be due to the fact that the patients who received it had a better original prognosis.

NON-RANDOMIZED STUDY

All patients receive the same investigational treatment.

PLACEBO STUDY

A placebo study has an inactive substance as one of its treatment arms. This type of study is used when no one knows if any treatment will be effective, or if other factors might be affecting results, such as a method of delivery. There are very few placebo studies for brain tumors. And, no study uses a placebo without informing patients that they might receive one.

CONTROL GROUP

Patients receiving standard treatment are called the control group.

DOUBLE-BLIND STUDY

In a double-blind study, neither the doctor nor the patient knows which drug is being given. In a single-blind study, the patients don't know which treatment they are receiving.

Finding and Evaluating
a Clinical Trial

Over two hundred clinical trials are available for brain tumor patients, and there is a profusion of information about them scattered among dozens of resources. Sorting through all that information can be challenging.

Be aware that not all sources have complete information. Some clinical trials may appear on one list and not another. And, some resources omit detail—entry criteria or phase number might be missing, for example. Some of these issues will be addressed by a new federal law which requires the inclusion of all clinical trials on a database to be maintained by the National Institutes of Health.

Some of the many sources currently available to you are listed below.

▲ Finding a trial

ASK YOUR DOCTORS

Your doctors might be investigators in a trial, or might know of trials for which you would qualify. They can perform a medical literature search looking for open clinical trials, or contact colleagues in the field. Your doctors can assist you in interpreting the information you obtain on your own. They can help you determine if a particular trial is appropriate for you and if you meet the entry criteria

Asking your doctor to help you look for a clinical trial, to follow up on your leads or to contact specialists at brain tumor referral centers is a reasonable request. Your doctor will not be insulted or think you are unduly demanding. And the specialists will be happy to provide whatever information they can about trials for which you might qualify, and outline the follow-up program for when you return home. Don't be shy or feel guilty about asking for help.

DO A PDQ SEARCH

Over 200 brain tumor clinical trials are listed in the National Cancer Institute's (NCI) *Physician Data Query* database. PDQ can be accessed by phone through the Cancer Information Service at (800) 422-6237 (800-4-CANCER). If you have access to the Internet, a version of PDQ is available at

http://cancertrials.nci.nih.gov or
http://cancernet.nci.nih.gov

Both databases include information about entry criteria for each of the clinical trials they list.

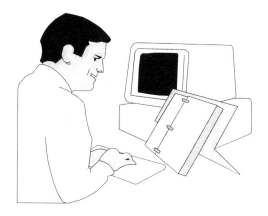

AL MUSELLA'S LIST of CLINICAL TRIALS and NOTEWORTHY TREATMENTS for BRAIN TUMORS .
This is an extensive listing of brain tumor protocols and information compiled and maintained on the Internet by Al Musella, DPM. Access the list at **http://virtualtrials.com**

CANCERFAX

NCI offers **CancerFax**, a cancer information database that can be searched using your fax machine. CancerFax can be reached by calling **(301) 402-5874** from your fax phone. If this is the first time you are using the CancerFax system, choose the option of printing a menu. An extensive range of information can be retrieved through this fax program. If you don't have a fax, the same information can be mailed to you by the Cancer Information Service.

CENTERWATCH

CenterWatch Clinical Trials Listing Service™ is available at **http://www.centerwatch.com** The trials are listed by pharmaceutical companies and physicians conducting research at major medical centers and private research centers.

Contact the NATIONAL INSTITUTE of NEUROLOGIC DISORDERS and STROKE

The National Institute of Neurologic Disorders and Stroke (NINDS) can be reached at **(800) 352-9424.** NINDS conducts clinical trials at the National Institutes of Health in Bethesda, Maryland.

AMERICAN BRAIN TUMOR ASSOCIATION

Call us at **(800) 886-2282.** We have a nationwide listing of doctors participating in clinical trials funded by the National Cancer Institute / National Institutes of Health. We can also provide information about some of the clinical trials sponsored by hospitals or pharmaceutical companies. In addition, we maintain a list of Internet sites that offer information about clinical trials and various other topics.

▲ Evaluating a trial

If you are considering a specific clinical trial, we encourage you to seek out as much information as is available about that new treatment. Because Phase I trials are just beginning their testing, little might be published about them. On the other hand, a considerable amount of information is available by the time a trial reaches Phase III.

BEGIN BY SPEAKING WITH THE INVESTIGATOR

The investigator is the doctor who explains the details of the trial, enrolls you into the trial, is responsible for delivering the treatment, doing follow-up studies and making progress reports.

Suggested questions:
- When did the trial begin?
- How many people have been treated so far?
- How many patients have your type of tumor?
- How well are they doing?
- Where will the treatment take place? Can it be administered close to your home?
- How many treatments will there be? How long will each one take? What is the interval between treatments?
- What costs are involved? Will your health insurance cover it?
- What type of follow-up is specified by the study? Who will provide it?

The investigator can provide you with a copy of the **complete protocol** and the **informed consent form** so you can share the information with your family. The complete protocol provides information about how the treatment will be given, what medical tests are involved and how often they are required. The informed consent form includes information about the hoped-for benefits, known risks and reported side-effects of the new treatment. Be sure you read and understand it. Ask questions about anything that is unclear or that you are concerned about. Many clinical trial teams include a nurse who is knowledgeable about the protocol for that trial. The nurse can answer questions about the trial or provide you with literature about the new treatment.

SEARCH THE MEDICAL LITERATURE

Computerized search programs, such as Medline, can help you find abstracts of case reports or review articles. If you retrieve the actual articles, note the date the article was *submitted* for publication (this date appears near the end of the article). Additional patients might have been treated since then, or the results of the trial might have changed. Ask your doctor to update you and help you interpret the reports. Medline searches can be done online at **http://igm.nlm.nih.gov**, at some local libraries or a medical library.

OBTAIN RESULTS OF PREVIOUS PHASES OF THE TRIAL

These are available from the principal investigator or through a medical literature search. Again, remember that the information you find will be outdated because it is based only on the data available at the time the article was written.

If you participated in a clinical trial and would like to know the **outcome results**, contact the principal investigator. Several clinical cooperative groups make results available to participants requesting them.

Chapter 10

Side-Effects and Their Management

Brain tumor treatments affect normal cells as well as tumor cells. Side-effects are caused by the treatment's affect on normal cells. Some side-effects are minimal, causing only minor discomfort. Others can be serious. Since side-effects vary with each person, you may experience some and not others, or none at all.

In this chapter, we explain and offer suggestions for managing some of the more common side-effects. Your doctors and nurses can provide more specific guidance for coping with problems you encounter. You will probably receive a lot of information about your treatment. Your nurses can help you sort through and understand much of it. They can also guide you to the specialists within the healthcare system who can help you with specific problems. For instance, pharmacists can advise you about the potential side-effects of the medications you'll take at home and what reactions your doctor should know about immediately. Psychologists and other specialists can teach you complementary therapies, such as relaxation techniques, to help control treatment or disease-related effects. Social workers can link you to community resources with support services.

Radiation Therapy Side-Effects

There are several types of radiation therapy. The Radiation Therapy section in Chapter 8 describes most of them. Side-effects depend on the type of radiation you receive and the total dosage. Your physician and nurse can tell you which ones you are likely to experience. The following side-effects are relative to conventional radiation therapy.

▲ Hair loss

Hair loss will probably be the first side-effect you experience. It occurs about two weeks after you begin radiation therapy. Hair loss is usually over the area being treated, but some people lose all of their hair. Hair loss is sudden, and it usually falls out in clumps over a short period of time. This can be very upsetting unless you are prepared for it. Hair loss is usually temporary; your radiation oncologist can advise you about this. Your hair will begin to grow back within weeks to months following therapy, but the new growth might not

be the same texture or color as your original hair. Permanent hair loss over the area being treated can occur with higher doses of radiation.

Management of hair loss

To minimize hair loss, cut your hair short before you begin treatment. This reduces the weight on the hair shaft. Satin pillowcases help lessen tangling while you sleep. Use an infant comb and brush set when your hair begins to grow back. Don't over shampoo your hair. Use a mild shampoo, such as a baby shampoo. Don't use abusive products on your hair, such as hot rollers, curling irons, hair sprays or dyes.

Consider purchasing a wig, or buy some scarves, turbans or caps before starting radiation. You might be able to purchase a wig from your own hair stylist. Wigs can also be made from your own hair. Hair pieces and wigs might be tax-deductible or covered by your insurance. Get a prescription for a "cranial prosthesis" (wig) from your physician. Recently, specialty stores have been established to help persons undergoing therapy obtain a variety of items and devices to help make their treatment easier to endure. Ask your nurse, social worker or local cancer society representative if they can refer you to a store in your area.

▲ Skin irritation

During radiation, the skin in the area being treated can become reddened, flaky and itchy. Don't try to treat these problems by yourself. Notify your physician immediately of the irritation.

Management of skin irritation

There are several things you can do to try to **prevent** this side-effect. Use a mild shampoo when you wash your hair and limit your hair washing to two or three times a week at most. Don't use abrasive hair treatments, such as hot rollers, conditioners, hair sprays or dyes. **Don't use anything on your scalp unless your doctor approves it.** Lotions and oils may increase the irritation. Corn starch can be used to decrease itching, if approved by your physician.

Stay out of the sun as much as possible and wear a hat or scarf when you are outside. Don't use hot water bottles, icepacks or heating pads on your scalp. Don't use tape, gauze or bandages on your scalp unless your physician tells you it's okay to do so.

▲ Hearing problems

In addition to skin irritation, you might have some temporary hearing difficulties. This can be due to hardening of the wax in your ears if your ears are in or near the area being radiated. Notify your physician if you experience a decrease in your hearing.

▲ Nausea or vomiting

Nausea caused by radiation therapy isn't very common, but it can occur following a treatment session.

Management of nausea and vomiting

If you experience nausea and/or vomiting after a treatment session, your doctor might prescribe a medication called an antiemetic. These are generally very effective at minimizing or controlling nausea. Antiemetics can also be used for "anticipatory nausea"—if you feel sick to your stomach prior to treatment.

Relaxation, imagery and biofeedback are techniques which can be used with or without antiemetics, to help you control this side-effect. Ask your physician or nurse where you can learn about these methods.

Additional suggestions

▸ Relax. Don't assume you'll be sick.
▸ Avoid eating for a few hours before treatment, if you experience nausea following the sessions.
▸ Stay away from fatty or spicy foods, sweets and strong smelling foods.
▸ Ice chips; ginger ale; unsalted pretzels; plain crackers; and/or cool, bland foods can help combat nausea.
▸ Drink plenty of water.
▸ Plan to eat your meals when the nausea is least troublesome.

▲ Changes in appetite

Your appetite may increase or decrease during the course of treatment. Some people lose weight and continue to lose weight for several weeks after finishing their treatments. Others gain weight, usually due to the corticosteroids they are taking.

Management of appetite changes

Whether your appetite has increased or decreased, it is important to eat a balanced diet. Small frequent meals may be easier for you. Eat when you're hungry rather than at set mealtimes.

If you are losing weight, try adding nutritional supplements to milk shakes or malts. Eat what appeals to you. Have snacks handy to nibble on throughout the day. Liquids may be more tempting than solids.

Weight gain due to steroids is generally unavoidable. Watch what you eat; nibble on healthy foods such as celery or carrots. Choose lower calorie, lower fat foods, such as a chicken breast instead of hamburger. Most people lose weight once they no longer need to take steroids.

▲ Drowsiness and fatigue

Most people experience some degree of fatigue and drowsiness during radiation therapy. The severity of these symptoms depends on the state of your health before the treatment. See the special section on fatigue later in this chapter.

▲ Decreased sex drive (libido)

Desire for sexual activity might be lowered because your hormone levels are affected, because you are stressed, or because you are just too tired.

Management of decreased sex drive

Share your thoughts with your partner. Explain that this is a side-effect of treatment, not a change in your feelings, and that your sexual desires will likely return to normal once treatment ends. Now is a time for closeness: hold hands; spend quiet time together. If you or your partner is concerned, speak to a counselor or social worker.

▲ Neurologic (brain) effects

Potential side-effects of radiation therapy are classified into three groups: acute, early delayed (also called sub-acute), and late.

ACUTE REACTIONS

These reactions occur during or immediately after radiation is finished. They are caused by radiation-induced brain swelling.

Symptoms can mimic the symptoms of your brain tumor, like speech problems or muscle weakness; or those of increased intracranial pressure, such as headache, nausea, double vision.

Management of acute reactions

Acute reactions are temporary and are usually relieved by corticosteroids such as dexamethasone. Often, steroids are prescribed to be taken during the entire treatment so that acute side-effects are avoided or minimized. The steroid dose is gradually reduced and discontinued when treatment is completed. Steroids are discussed more fully in Chapter 12.

EARLY DELAYED (SUB-ACUTE) REACTIONS

This group of reactions occurs a few weeks to a few months after completion of therapy, most commonly between one and three months. Symptoms include loss of appetite, sleepiness, lack of energy, as well as an increase in pre-existing neurologic symptoms.

Some of these reactions are thought to be due to a temporary disruption of myelin formation (demyelination). Myelin is a substance which helps speed the relay of nerve signals. The symptoms are usually temporary—lasting about six weeks, the length of time it takes for myelin to repair itself. In some cases, however, recovery may take up to several months.

Since the brain lacks an effective lymph system, dead tumor cells are cleared away very slowly. A rapid build-up of dead cells can lead to swelling which might produce a temporary increase of symptoms. CT scans taken shortly after treatment might show changes that are difficult to distinguish from tumor growth. Repeat CT or MRI scans are often necessary to clarify the cause of the symptoms.

Management of early delayed reactions

Notify your radiation oncologist or your primary doctor if you notice any of the symptoms listed. Early delayed reactions are usually treated with steroids and most of these reactions are self-limiting—they go away with minimal treatment. However, they can become life-threatening if they aren't treated properly. Therefore, it's important for your doctors to be aware if you experience these reactions so they can monitor your progress and adjust your steroid medications, if necessary.

Leukoencephalopathy is a type of early delayed reaction affecting the white matter (connective tissue) of the brain. It occurs when the white matter is irritated by radiation, dead tumor cells, and/or other treatments, such as chemotherapy. The severity of the symptoms increases with the amount of damage. Leukoencephalopathy may be reversible and is usually treated with steroids.

LATE REACTIONS

These reactions are due to changes in the white matter and death of brain tissue caused by radiation-damaged blood vessels. Symptoms can occur months to years after therapy is completed. These long-term effects are permanent and can be progressive. Symptoms vary from mild to severe and include: decreased intellect, memory impairment, confusion, personality changes, and alteration of the normal function of the area irradiated.

It is sometimes difficult to diagnose late delayed reactions. CT and MRI scans might be unable to distinguish between new tumor growth and radiation changes. PET scanning might be helpful, but is not totally accurate either. A biopsy of the area might be the only way to determine whether you have radiation changes to your brain or new tumor growth.

Management of late delayed reactions

Mild reactions may be treated with steroids. Severe reactions such as tumor necrosis may require surgery to remove the dead tissue. This need for surgery is common in patients who receive very high doses of radiation, such as that used during interstitial radiation or radiosurgery. Research into preventing this type of injury is underway.

▲ Other reactions

▸ **Oncogenesis**, the development of another tumor, is now a recognized, although rare, possible long-term side-effect of radiation.

▸ Radiation therapy might also cause **pituitary-hypothalamic dysfunction** (changes in normal hormone levels) leading to problems with your thyroid, sugar metabolism, fertility, or ability to process water.

▸ Because their brains are still developing, **children** are extremely susceptible to the side-effects of radiation. Treatment with radiation is delayed as long as possible, or at least until a child is three years old.

Recent research has focused on the long-term effects of radiation in children. These include physical consequences, and psychological, social and educational effects as well. Information about this research can be obtained through medical literature searches, such as Medline.

Chemotherapy Side-Effects

Chemotherapy drugs affect all cells—tumor cells as well as normal ones. The side-effects you experience are the result of the drug's affect on normal, actively dividing cells. The faster cells divide, the more sensitive they are to chemotherapy. Some of the fastest dividing cells in your body are bone marrow—the part of the body that makes new blood cells; the cells that line the stomach, mouth and intestines; and hair cells. That is why they are the most commonly affected cells. Chemotherapy may also affect organs such as your liver.

Normal cells are capable of repairing themselves following chemotherapy, while tumor cells have a limited ability to do so. The goal of chemotherapy is to give enough drug to kill tumor cells without causing permanent damage to normal cells. The amount of chemotherapy that can safely be given to a patient is based on that drug's potential to damage normal tissue—*drug toxicity*.

The severity of side-effects varies with the type of drug, how it is given, how much is given, and one's general health. When your doctor talks with you and your family about chemotherapy, ask about the potential side-effects of the drugs you will be receiving. Your doctor can put them into perspective and help you weigh the risks against the benefits.

————————

The following are some points to consider when you discuss chemotherapy.

▸ Side-effects are drug specific; that is, certain side-effects are associated with certain drugs. For example, some chemotherapy drugs cause hair-loss and others do not.

▸ Side-effects vary with each individual. While you might experience a side-effect, someone else taking the same drug may not.

▸ Some side-effects occur during or immediately after the drug is given. Other side-effects are delayed and might not occur for days or weeks.

▸ Most side-effects are reversible when chemotherapy is ended.

▸ The drug dose can be modified by your doctor if the side-effects become uncomfortable.

▸ The decision to have chemotherapy is **not** a permanent one. If you change your mind, tell your doctor. Your treatment can be changed, modified or stopped completely. Discuss other options with your doctor.

▸ There are many successful methods of preventing or managing the side-effects of chemotherapy. Ask your doctor or nurse about new anti-nausea drugs, imaging and relaxation techniques and other coping tactics.

▲ Effects on bone marrow

Blood cells are produced by bone marrow. If the marrow is affected, the production of blood cells is also affected.

RED BLOOD CELLS (RBCs) —————————

Red blood cells carry oxygen to all parts of your body. When you don't have enough red blood cells in your system, you are *anemic*. Anemia might cause you to feel tired, dizzy or chilly, or become short of breath. You may also look pale.

Management of low red blood cell counts

▸ Get plenty of rest, and eat a well-balanced diet.

▸ Eat foods that are high in iron such as green leafy vegetables.

▸ Don't be embarrassed or reluctant to ask for help when you need it.

▸ When you get up after sitting or lying down, move slowly and take deep breaths to avoid getting dizzy.

▸ Anemia may also contribute to a feeling of fatigue. See the special section on Fatigue later in this chapter.

Your doctor will check your red blood cell count regularly during treatment. If you experience severe anemia, medications can be prescribed to boost the production of red blood cells or a blood transfusion may be suggested.

WHITE BLOOD CELLS (WBCs) —————————

White blood cells fight infection. If your WBCs are low, you are at risk for an infection. An infection in someone with too few WBCs can be life-threatening. Common symptoms of an infection include fever, chills, sweating, diarrhea, sore throat, cough, mouth sores or burning while urinating. If a cut or wound becomes red, swollen or has drainage, it is probably infected. Notify your doctor immediately if you think you have any kind of an infection.

Management of low white blood cell counts

The best way to combat infection is to prevent it. *To prevent infection:*

▸ Wash your hands often, especially before eating and after using the bathroom. Wash your hands after handling pets. Make sure those who are helping you wash their hands also.

▸ Get plenty of rest, avoid fatigue, eat a well-balanced diet.

▸ Practice good oral hygiene. Use soft toothbrushes and brush gently.

▸ Wash all fresh fruits and vegetables thoroughly before eating them.

- Avoid crowds.
- Avoid persons who are ill. Tell them they can't visit you until they have recovered.
- Avoid children who have recently received immunization shots. Don't get any immunization shots yourself.
- Use lotion to prevent your hands from becoming dry or cracked.
- Be careful not to cut yourself when using a knife or razor. Use an electric razor for shaving.
- Clean cuts or other wounds immediately with warm water and soap.
- Use protective gloves when washing dishes or gardening. Use potholders or gloves when cooking.
- It's best to have someone else clean up after pets. If that's not possible, use gloves and wash your hands thoroughly afterward.

Your physician will check your white blood count regularly during treatment. If it falls too low, medications to boost the production of WBCs might be prescribed. If your count becomes dangerously low you may need to be hospitalized.

PLATELETS
Platelets are the cells that help stop bleeding by forming blood clots. If your platelets are low, you bruise more easily and it takes longer for cuts and scrapes to stop bleeding. Other symptoms of a low platelet count include small, red spots on your skin, pink-tinged to red urine, bloody or black stools, and bleeding from the gums or nose. Women may experience heavier than normal menstrual bleeding.

Management of low platelet counts:
Notify your doctor immediately if you experience any of the symptoms listed. Avoid medications that enhance bleeding, such as aspirin, ibuprofen and other anti-inflammatories. If you are unsure if you can take a medication, ask your doctor or pharmacist.

Try to avoid activities that can cause injury. Use work gloves and protective gear when gardening or doing other work that can lead to cuts or scrapes. Check with your doctor before participating in sports activities such as football, rollerblading, biking, etc. Try not to blow your nose too hard, cough too harshly or strain at bowel movements.

If you cut yourself, put pressure on the wound for 10 to 15 minutes. If the bleeding doesn't stop, notify your doctor. If you suffer a major injury, go to the nearest emergency room.

Your doctor will check your platelet count regularly during treatment. If it is too low, you may require a transfusion.

▲ Effects on the digestive system
The digestive system includes the **mouth, esophagus, stomach and intestines**. Inflammation of the cells lining these organs is called *mucositis*.

MOUTH AND ESOPHAGUS
Mucositis in the mouth is called *stomatitis*; in the esophagus, it is called *esophagitis*. Mucositis usually begins with a dry mouth, tongue and lips. Burning or tingling sensations may also occur. This may make chewing and swallowing uncomfortable.

Notify your doctor immediately if you develop any sores or ulcers in your mouth or if swallowing becomes painful.

Management of mouth and esophagus problems
Prevention
Good oral hygiene is extremely important for the prevention of mucositis.
- Brush your teeth with a soft toothbrush after meals and at bedtime.
- Floss regularly with unwaxed dental floss.
- Gargle with salt water or a mouthwash that contains no alcohol. Baking soda in water is another good mouth rinse, but some people don't like the taste.
- Hydrogen peroxide and water should not be used unless your doctor instructs you to do so.

▶ Remember to remove dentures so the gums can be washed and rinsed.

▶ Don't use lemon glycerin swabs—they dry out the mouth and might decalcify your teeth.

▶ Avoid alcoholic drinks. Don't smoke.

▶ Moisten your lips with lip ointment or water-soluble lubricating jelly.

▶ Use sugarless candy or gum if your mouth is dry. Different types of artificial saliva are available. Ask your doctor, nurse or pharmacist for their recommendations.

▶ Drink plenty of water.

▶ Avoid citrus fruits and juices and other acid containing foods. Avoid spicy foods.

If you develop sores in your mouth

▶ Notify your doctor.

▶ Eat bland foods at moderate temperatures.

▶ Moisten dry foods.

▶ Eat soft foods or foods prepared in a blender.

▶ Try milkshakes, applesauce and soft non-citrus fruits, mashed potatoes, scrambled eggs, puddings and gelatin.

▶ Use a topical anesthetic for mouth sores, available at your drug store.

▶ Use frozen popsicles, ice chips or other frozen foods to relieve mouth pain.

STOMACH AND INTESTINES

Diarrhea **or** constipation can occur if your intestines (bowels) are affected. Symptoms can begin one to six hours after chemotherapy and might last a few hours, several days, or a few weeks.

People assume they will have nausea and vomiting during chemotherapy. This is **not** always the case. This side-effect is highly dependent on the type of drug used, and many drugs used for primary brain tumors do not cause nausea and vomiting.

Antinausea medications, called *antiemetics*, help stop or limit nausea and vomiting. Your doctor will discuss these medicines with you when planning your chemotherapy.

Management of nausea and vomiting

▶ Relax. Don't assume you will be sick.

▶ Use imaging and other relaxation techniques before and during your therapy. Biofeedback, self-hypnosis, diversionary activities (videos, games, puzzles), accu-pressure and music therapy may be helpful.

▶ Avoid eating for a few hours before treatment, if you experience nausea.

▶ Stay away from fatty or spicy foods, sweets and strong smelling foods.

▶ Ice chips, ginger ale, unsalted pretzels, plain crackers, cool, bland foods can help combat nausea.

▶ Try small, frequent meals. Eat slowly.

▶ Have your favorite foods available and located conveniently.

▶ Drink plenty of water.

Management of constipation

Prevention is the best medicine.

▶ Drink plenty of fluids.

▶ Eat bulky, high-fiber foods such as bran and whole wheat products.

▶ Exercise daily, if possible—even a short walk is helpful in preventing constipation.

Notify your doctor if you are troubled by this side-effect. Medications can be prescribed.

Management of diarrhea

▶ Drink plenty of fluids to prevent becoming dehydrated. Fluids high in electrolytes, such as Pedialyte, are preferable. Sports drinks, such as Gatorade, may be suggested. Plain water, weak tea or apple juice can also be helpful.

▶ Eat high calorie, high protein, low residue foods.

▶ Eat small, frequent meals. Eat bland foods.

▶ Avoid foods at temperature extremes—hot or cold.

▶ While you have diarrrhea, avoid high-fiber foods and foods that can irritate the bowel: bran, whole grain breads, fried foods, fruit juices, milk products, coffee, etc.

▸ Avoid gas-producing foods such as onions, cabbage, beans etc. Artificial sweeteners cause gas in some people.

▸ Dietary supplements such as Ensure and Sustacal may contribute to diarrhea. Avoid using these products until your diarrhea is under control.

▸ If you can tolerate them, eat foods high in potassium, such as cantaloupe, oranges, peaches, bananas and baked potatoes.

▸ Use mild soap and water to wash your anal area; pat dry. Sitz baths can be soothing.

▸ Use moisture barrier creams and ointments, such as A&D ointment or Desitin if your skin becomes irritated. Notify your physician if you develop any sores.

▲ Skin reactions

Chemotherapy can cause minor skin reactions such as rash, itching, dryness or acne.

Notify your doctor immediately if you develop a sudden rash or hives, severe itching, shortness of breath or wheezing. These are indications of an allergic reaction that needs to be treated immediately. In extreme cases, this type of reaction constitutes a medical emergency.

Management of skin reactions

▸ Wash with a mild, unperfumed soap or skin lotion. Look for hypoallergenic soaps. Softer soaps such as Dove and Neutrogena are closer to your skin's normal pH and will not cause dryness.

▸ Avoid perfumes, perfumed lotions and products that contain alcohol. Alcohol is drying to your skin.

▸ Use warm, **not hot**, water for bathing. Pat your skin dry rather than rubbing.

▸ Cornstarch patted on the skin may relieve itching. (Don't use talc.)

▸ Some chemotherapy medications cause you to sunburn more easily. Check with your doctor to see if you should use a heavy duty sun screen when you are outdoors.

▸ If chemotherapy is given through a vein, some skin discoloration might occur along the path of the vein. The darkened area usually fades when treatment ends.

▲ Hair loss

Some chemotherapy drugs cause hair loss; others do not. Ask your doctor if you can expect this side-effect from the chemotherapy you will be receiving.

Hair loss due to chemotherapy isn't permanent; your hair will grow back after your therapy is completed.

Management of hair loss

To minimize hair loss, cut your hair short before you begin treatment. This reduces the weight on the hair shaft. Satin pillowcases help lessen tangling while you sleep. Use an infant comb and brush set when your hair begins to grow back. Don't over shampoo your hair. Use a mild shampoo which is "pH balanced," such as a baby shampoo. Don't use abusive products on your hair, such as hot rollers, curling irons, hair sprays or dyes.

Consider purchasing a wig or buy some scarves, turbans or caps before starting radiation. You might be able to purchase a wig from your hair stylist. Wigs can also be made from your own hair. Hair pieces and wigs might be tax-deductible or covered by your insurance. Get a prescription for a "cranial prosthesis" (wig) from your physician. Recently, specialty stores have been established to help persons undergoing therapy obtain a variety of items and devices to help make their treatment easier to endure. Ask your nurse or local cancer society representative if they can refer you to a store in your area.

Fatigue

Fatigue is a symptom experienced by almost everyone undergoing treatment for a brain tumor. Fatigue related to tumors is different from the fatigue you might have experienced in the past. This type of fatigue is more severe, persistent, and not necessarily the result of physical activity. It can be unpredictable and emotionally over-whelming. Most telling, it isn't fully relieved by rest or sleep. In this section, we will discuss the probable causes of tumor-related fatigue and offer some suggestions for battling this debilitating symptom.

▲ Causes of fatigue

Many factors contribute to the fatigue experienced by brain tumor patients. First is the emotional impact of receiving the diagnosis of a brain tumor. Surgery is an assault to your body and causes fatigue. Radiation and chemotherapy can cause fatigue by adding a new task to your already full, daily routine. Treatments may make you feel ill, and side-effects are stressful to both your body and your emotions.

Your sleep cycle might be disturbed in several ways. First, you may need to take medications during the night. Your sleep may be disturbed by the side-effects of treatments, such as urinary frequency, nausea, cramps, diarrhea, etc. You may also be disturbed by well-meaning friends and family who call to find out how you are when you are trying to rest.

Fatigue can also be caused by the cell-killing effects of treatment. Your body is hard-at-work removing damaged cells and waste. This alone might be tiring.

There is no quick fix for this type of fatigue; sleep alone doesn't solve the problem. You will need to re-prioritize your activities and manage normal, everyday tasks in a new way. This in itself is a cause of fatigue. Keep a diary of what you are doing to combat fatigue: what seems to help and what doesn't; what makes you more fatigued and what brings relief.

▲ Self-care

These are the routine, daily activities you perform to prepare and care for yourself during the day. Your nurse, occupational therapist and physical therapist are good resources for hints on how to make self-care easier.

▸ Become very organized: Lay out your clothes ahead of time (or have someone else do it for you, if need be). Organize toiletries so they are all in a single, convenient place. Use a shower or bath organizer so you don't have to bend or reach while bathing. Avoid rushing.

▸ Use assistive devices, such as grab rails in the bathroom, a raised toilet seat, extension handles on brushes and sponges, to minimize the energy you need to expend.

▸ Use a shower chair to bathe. Sit down to dry off. Avoid bending and leaning over as much as possible.

▸ Organize your home to be as efficient as possible. The closer things are to each other, the less energy you need to spend on getting to them.

▸ Wear comfortable clothes and low-heeled shoes.

▲ Activities

On a daily basis, you participate in many activities: work, leisure, household tasks, child care, etc. If possible, let others help you by assuming some of your responsibilities. Allow people to cook, clean your home or shop for you. It may be difficult and a little stressful for you to give up some of your independence, but in the long run it will help you.

▸ Organize your time. Schedule those activities that are the most important to you during the times when you have the most energy. Pace yourself and don't overdo it.

▸ If you have a lot of helpers, take advantage of them. You may want to assign one person to organize the others and assign their tasks.

▸ When you do housework, sit down whenever possible. Schedule tasks throughout the week instead of doing them all at once. Delegate housework as much as possible.

▸ When shopping, organize your list by store aisle. Shop when it's less busy so you don't have to wait in line to be checked out. Ask someone to help load the groceries into your car. Delegate shopping whenever possible.

▸ When preparing meals, sit down as much as possible. Prepare double amounts and freeze half. Soak dishes instead of scrubbing; let dishes air dry. Use the dishwasher as much as possible. Delegate cooking and clean-up as much as possible.

▸ Child care is a difficult issue, because young children may not understand why you can't spend as much time with them as you used to. Plan activities that allow you to sit and at a time when you have the most energy. Try to explain your limitations; answer their questions truthfully, but at a level they can understand. Teach your children to climb onto your lap, rather than expecting you to lift them. Have someone help with activities involving lifting.

▲ Sleep, rest and exercise

Rest is extremely important to your battle with fatigue. It is also one of the hardest things to do.

NIGHT TIME TIPS

▸ Decrease environmental noise: close windows, use a white noise machine. Tell family members that you are going to bed and ask them to keep noise to a minimum. Turn off the phone in your bedroom and let the answering machine pick up any calls.

▸ Go to bed at about the same time every day. Develop a sleep routine. Let friends know what time you go to sleep so they won't call you.

▸ Don't eat or drink anything with caffeine late in the day. Try herbal teas or decaffeinated coffees. Avoid chocolate.

▸ Don't drink too much late in the day, unless it's necessary during your treatments.

▸ Avoid taking sleeping pills, if possible. They can disrupt your normal sleep cycle and you will feel groggy the next day.

NAPPING & RESTING TIPS

▸ Take a short nap during the day. Naps are good, but make sure they aren't too long or so late in the day that they interfere with your nighttime sleep.

▸ Allow yourself some quiet time each day. Remove yourself from others and spend it in a peaceful place. Walk in a natural environment such as a park or garden. Spend time in activities that interest you to take your mind off your treatments. "Time off" helps you gain energy.

▸ Investigate meditation, self-guided imagery, music therapy, yoga and other complementary treatments.

EXERCISE

▸ Try to fit an activity such as walking into your daily schedule. Exercise promotes a healthier body and helps reduce psychological stress. Exercise may also help you sleep better at night.

▸ Don't overdo your exercise routine. Ask your physical therapist to help you develop a routine. Increase activity gradually. If you do too much all at once, you'll increase your fatigue.

Chapter 11

Complementary and Alternative Medicine

Many complementary and alternative therapies date back to ancient cultures whose management of disease was based on spirituality, prayer, herbal remedies and acupuncture. Modern Eastern cultures continue to use these therapies far more commonly than Western cultures. Therapies called "alternative" in the US may be called "complementary" in Europe. Complementary treatments such as acupuncture and herbalism are traditional medicine in Asia.

In a search for less toxic therapies and improved quality of life, increasing numbers of patients are turning to complementary and alternative treatments. Recent studies reveal that about 50% of cancer patients in the United States are using some form of these therapies, often without the knowledge of their doctors.

Complementary and Alternative Medicine refers to a broad range of therapies used both to treat and prevent disease. Practitioners of complementary and alternative medicine believe that the state of your health is dependent on the whole you: your body, your mind and your spirit. This holistic approach is the foundation of many of these therapies.

The Terminology

» **Conventional medicine** is the mainstream medical care practiced at most hospitals in the US. Standards of care are set by government and regulatory agencies. In conventional medicine, an *effective cancer treatment* is defined as one that causes the size of a tumor to measurably shrink or remain stable.

» **Complementary medicine** is used *in addition to* conventional treatments. Cancer patients use these therapies primarily to manage or prevent pain, nausea, and treatment related side-effects; to reduce stress and anxiety; and to promote healing. Complementary therapies can relieve symptoms and improve the quality of life for some patients. Other names for complementary medicine are *holistic medicine* and *natural medicine*.

» **Alternative medicine** is often used *instead of* conventional treatments. Many alternative therapies seek to treat illness by helping the body to heal itself or to treat the "source" of the disease.

» **Integrative medicine** combines conventional medical care with complementary and/or alternative therapies. Chiropractic care, acupuncture, herbal medicine, massage therapy, behavioral therapies, and mind-body self-care are often integrated with conventional treatment.

Types of Therapy

Listed below are some of the many therapies of interest to cancer patients. For more information, use the resources listed at the end of this chapter.

acupressure	acupuncture
antineoplastons	antioxidants
aromatherapy	biofeedback
crystal therapy	energy balancing
Essiac tea	expressive therapy
	art, music, dance, etc.

green tea	herbal remedies
homeopathy	hydrazine sulfate
imagery	massage therapy
magnet therapy	melatonin
meditation	nutritional therapies
reflexology	relaxation techniques
shark cartilage	shiatsu
spirituality	St. John's wort
therapeutic touch	visualization
yoga	

Seeking a Complementary or Alternative Therapy

▲ Research the treatment

Information about these therapies is available in books, from organizations supporting their use, on the Internet and from friends and family. Learn as much as you can from as many resources as possible. Don't rely on one book, one magazine article or one disciple. Look for the source's credentials—Is the author licensed? What is his or her educational background, professional society affiliations? Your research will help you make an educated decision.

Be cautious with any therapy claiming to have no side-effects. For example, natural herbs have side-effects and contraindications just like prescription medicines. The essential oils used for aromatherapy may be beneficial when used as directed, but can be poisonous if swallowed.

▲ Finding a practitioner

Several major hospitals now offer Integrative Medicine centers. Find out if your hospital is one of them. Complementary therapies may be offered by your hospital's Cancer Center or in the Behavioral Medicine department.

Your doctor may be able to refer you to a practitioner. Or, determine if there is a professional organization for practitioners of the therapy in which you are interested. If there is, obtain a list of their members. Several of the resources listed below can help you find out about professional organizations.

Inquire about the background and training of the practitioner. Does their specialty offer certification and if so, is he or she certified? Some states require licensing of practitioners, such as naturopaths and acupuncturists. Find out if the practitioner has the credentials to practice the treatment.

▲ Use reasonable caution

There might be little or no documented evidence from clinical studies of the full effects of these therapies. Before you pursue any form of complementary or alternative medicine, let your doctor know what you want to do so you can be sure the new therapy does not adversely affect or interfere with any of your current treatments. For example, large doses of antioxidants might make radiation therapy less effective. Share the information you obtained about the therapy with your physician—how the substance is used, how it works, known side-effects and contraindications. Together, if appropriate, you can incorporate the therapy into your treatment plan.

Reading Materials

Collinge, William. *The American Holistic Health Association's Complete Guide to Alternative Medicine.* Warner Books. 1996. ISBN 0-446-67258-0. Principles of the treatments, variations, techniques, how to choose a practitioner including licensing, certification and training information, costs, and how to evaluate results.

Duke, James A. *The Green Pharmacy.* St. Martin's Press, 1997. ISBN 0-312-96648-2. Focuses on herbal remedies, includes explanations of their bio-chemical functions and uses.

Fugh-Berman, Adriane. *Alternative Medicine: What Works. A comprehensive, easy-to-read review of the scientific evidence, pro and con.* Odonian Press, Tucson, AZ. 1996. ISBN 1-878825-55-0. Results of clinical trials, controlled trials, and scientific literature references for alternative treatments. One of the few references focusing on scientific evaluation.

Goldberg, Burton. *Alternative Medicine. The Definitive Guide.* Future Medicine Publishing, Inc. Tiburon, CA. 1997. ISBN 0-9636334-3-0. A comprehensive guide compiled by over 300 alternative medicine practitioners includes statements of philosophy, political background information, how and why the various therapies are used, organizations offering additional information, and recommended readings.

Lerner, Michael. *Choices in Healing: Integrating the Best of Conventional and Complementary Approaches to Cancer.* The MIT Press, Cambridge, MA. 1994. ISBN 0-262-12180-8. An overview of complementary and alternative therapies, what they are, how they work, and how to learn more.

Nixon, Daniel. *The Cancer Recovery Eating Plan: The Right Foods to Help Fuel Your Recovery.* Times Book/Random House, New York, NY. 1996. ISBN 0-8129-2590-4. Easy healthful recipes for cancer survivors wishing to "maximize their recovery." The recipes incorporate familiar food items readily available in your kitchen or grocery.

Spiller, Gene; Bruce, Bonnie. *Cancer Survivor's Nutrition and Health Guide. Eating Well and Getting Better During and After Cancer Treatment.* Prima Publishing, Rocklin, CA. 1997. ISBN 0-7615-0581-4. Offers nutritional guidance for specific types of cancer, help with food substitutions, explanation of food labeling, and recipes.

Weil, Andrew. *Spontaneous Healing. How to Discover and Enhance Your Body's Natural Ability to Maintain and Heal Itself.* Ballatine Books, New York, NY. 1995. ISBN 0-449091064-4. Advocates the use of complementary and alternative therapies without abandoning conventional therapy, focuses on the ability of the mind to assist in healing the body.

For More Information

National Center for Complementary and Alternative Medicine (NCCAM)
National Institutes of Health
P. O. Box 8218
Silver Spring, MD 20907-8218
(888) 644-6226 (Toll free)
Fax (301) 495-4957
http://altmed.od.nih.gov

University of Texas Center for Alternative Medicine
http://www.sph.uth.tmc.edu/utcam
This is the only NCCAM supported institution focused solely on alternative and complementary treatments for cancer. The UT-CAM web site offers an extensive list of resources, organizations and links to alternative medicine web sites.

Inclusion in this chapter does not constitute endorsement of any author, method, treatment or philosophy.

Chapter 12

Steroids

Steroids are drugs used to reduce the edema (swelling) associated with brain tumors and their treatment. Dexamethasone (Decadron), prednisolone, and prednisone are examples of these drugs. Steroids can temporarily relieve symptoms, improve your neurological status, and promote a feeling of well-being. Long-term use is for relief of symptoms. Because of the potential side-effects of this class of drugs, long-term use requires close monitoring.

When steroids are discontinued, the amounts must be tapered slowly to allow time for your body to adjust. Your doctor will give you a detailed schedule for decreasing the dosage. Because steroids often "mask" symptoms, it is not unusual to experience those symptoms again when the steroids are discontinued.

Edema

Edema—swelling due to the accumulation of fluids in the tissue around a tumor—is common in brain tumor patients. It may be caused by the tumor itself or be a side-effect of surgery, radiation, or other forms of treatment. Edema can lead to increased intracranial pressure which, in turn, causes headaches and drowsiness. Steroids are medications used to reduce edema.

Dexamethasone (Decadron) and prednisone are commonly prescribed steroids.

Steroids and Surgery

Steroids may be given before and during surgery and are continued for several days after to control swelling caused by the operation. If edema is present before the surgery, high dose steroids may be started even earlier. Typically, steroid doses are tapered until they are discontinued during the week (or more) following surgery.

Steroids and Radiation Therapy

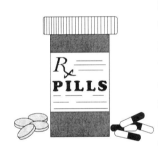

Steroids are often used to treat the early acute reactions to radiation therapy (those which occur during the course of treatment). Initially, steroids are taken every day, then their dose is decreased during, or at the end of, treatment depending on the radiation dosage schedule.

Steroids and Tumor-Caused Edema

The blood brain barrier, disrupted by the tumor, allows fluids to leak from small blood vessels and pool in the tissue around the tumor. This results in edema. Steroids quickly reduce edema by decreasing the leakiness of the blood brain barrier. The result is a rapid improvement of symptoms.

For patients with **recurrent tumors**, steroids can help improve the quality of their life by reducing symptoms without affecting alertness or the ability to communicate and interact with others.

Some types of tumors are particularly responsive to steroids, although it is unclear whether the drugs affect the tumor itself, or only the associated edema.

» To reduce the severe symptoms that can accompany **metastatic** brain tumors, the first treatment is often a course of steroid therapy. The drugs might eliminate the need for emergency surgery if the high level of intracranial pressure usually present can be controlled.

» If a **lymphoma** is suspected, steroid therapy is often delayed until the diagnosis is confirmed. These tumors are extremely sensitive to steroids and lymphomas have been known to disappear completely from scans following the use of these drugs. Rather than controlling edema, steroids are thought to actually destroy lymphoma tumor cells, but are not a cure for this tumor.

Side-Effects of Steroids

Steroids have several beneficial effects. They can:
▸ decrease symptoms dramatically
▸ promote a sense of well-being
▸ improve neurological status

Steroids also cause a wide range of side-effects that must be carefully monitored by your doctor.

The most common side-effects are: extreme weight gain due to water retention, causing a puffy, moon-shaped face; an increased appetite; and mood fluctuations. Other, more serious, side-effects can occur although they are less common.

The lowest **effective** dosage of steroid medications is always the goal.

The benefits of steroid use almost always outweigh their potential side-effects.

Managing Common Side-Effects

Steroids can cause **stomach irritation**. They should be taken with meals or with an antacid that your doctor prescribes for you. Be sure to call your doctor if you have stomach pains or run a temperature.

While taking steroids, you might experience **depression, mood swings, irritability, agitation, and/or sleep difficulties**. These symptoms are due to the steroid's effect on the natural hormone balance in your body. These side-effects can be treated and should be reported to your doctor. It is also helpful to discuss these effects with your family so they know what to expect and can be supportive. Talking about your feelings will also remind them that not all of your emotional reactions are caused by medications.

If you are **gaining water weight** from the steroids, controlling your appetite is even more important. Try to find low-calorie, low-salt foods to nibble between meals. Fresh-cut vegetable sticks or fresh fruit can often satisfy your appetite and not add more pounds.

Remember that steroids should never be stopped suddenly. Don't change your dose unless the doctor tells you to do so. When the steroids are stopped, they must be slowly withdrawn on a tapering schedule prescribed by your doctor. Since steroids do not kill tumor tissue, symptoms relieved by the tumor might begin again as the dosage is reduced.

Chapter 13

Seizures

Seizures are common symptoms of a brain tumor. For some people, a seizure may be the first clue that something unusual is happening in their brain.

Seizures might be caused by a brain tumor or the surgery to remove it. Seizures can also be totally unrelated to a brain tumor. For example, an injury to the head, a stroke, alcohol or drug withdrawal and fever can all cause seizures. Or, the cause may be unknown.

About 60% of all brain tumor patients will experience a seizure at least once during their illness. Seizures are particularly common with slow growing gliomas, meningiomas located in the convexity of the brain, and with metastatic brain tumors. Sometimes, seizures help alert the doctor to the presence of a tumor.

Most seizures can be controlled with medications called antiepileptics. It is important to tell your doctor if your seizures and/or the medications affect your quality of life. Your doctor will work with you to find the best medication to control your seizures and keep side-effects to a minimum.

What Are Seizures?

Seizures are sudden attacks that cause a wide range of unusual behaviors and sensations. They are due to abnormal electrical activity in the cerebral hemispheres of the brain. Normally, your body's nerve cells communicate with each other via carefully controlled electric signals. If something interferes with those signals and they become more intense, a seizure results. While seizures are usually brief, their effects may linger for several hours.

There are different types of seizures. The type you experience depends on which area of the brain has the abnormal electrical signals.

Most seizures occur randomly, at any time and without any particular cause. However, you might have some advance notice. Headache, mood changes and/or muscle jerking might signal a coming seizure. Those warning signals are called *auras*. An aura may precede a seizure by a few seconds or even minutes. Use that time to safeguard yourself. For example, if you are chewing, remove the food from your mouth. If you are walking, sit or lie down.

If you have recurrent seizures, you might notice that some events "trigger" them. Bright lights, flashing lights, specific odors, lack of sleep, missed meals, menses, increased stress or emotional difficulties, alcohol, new medications, or changed dosages of existing medications can all be triggers. Keeping track of what you were doing immediately prior to each seizure can help you identify your personal triggers. Having a seizure does not necessarily mean your tumor is growing.

A **seizure** is an attack caused by abnormal electrical activity in the brain. It lasts only a short period of time and may cause unusual movements, a change in the level or loss of consciousness, and/or sensory distortions. **Epilepsy** is defined as recurrent seizures.

Types of Seizures

There are two primary types of seizures—partial (also called focal) seizures and generalized seizures.

▲ Partial (Focal) Seizures

Partial seizures affect one part of a cerebral hemisphere. Symptoms depend on the part of the brain involved. Partial seizures may become generalized later in the attack. There are two types of partial seizures: **Simple partial seizures,** which don't cause unconsciousness and **complex partial seizures,** which do cause loss of consciousness.

▸ **Simple partial seizures** commonly cause convulsive jerking or twitching (if the frontal lobe is involved), tingling or numbness (if the parietal lobe is involved) or other unusual sensations. These symptoms can begin in one part of the body and then spread to other areas. Chewing movements or lip smacking (if the anterior temporal lobe is involved), buzzing in the ears, flashes of lights, sweating, flushing and pupil dilation are other common symptoms. Psychic symptoms include a sense of déjà vu; imaginary sights (if the occipital lobe is involved), smells (if the temporal lobe is involved) or tastes; or imaginary sounds.

▸ **Complex partial seizures** cause some loss of consciousness and usually indicate temporal lobe involvement. Purposeless, automatic movements might occur. The seizure may be preceded, accompanied or followed by psychic symptoms. A state of confusion may last for a time after the attack. In patients with low-grade gliomas, this is the most common type of seizure.

▲ Generalized seizures

These seizures may begin as partial seizures and abruptly change into generalized seizures. There are several different types of generalized seizures.

▸ **Absence (petit mal) seizures** cause an impairment of consciousness and may be accompanied by a feeling of limpness. The patient may miss a few words or stop speaking for a few seconds during a conversation. You may think he or she has been daydreaming. The beginning and end of the attack is usually sudden. This type of seizure most commonly begins in childhood and often stops by age 20.

▸ **Atypical absence seizures** may cause more extensive changes in muscle tone, or they may have a more gradual beginning and ending than typical absence seizures.

▸ **Atonic seizures,** also called *epileptic drop attacks,* are characterized by sudden limpness. Generally, all muscle tone and consciousness are lost.

▸ **Myoclonic seizures** cause single or multiple muscle twitches, jerks or spasms.

▸ **Tonic-clonic (grand mal) seizures** are common in people with low grade gliomas but can occur with all gliomas. The seizure begins with a sudden outburst and then a loss of consciousness. This is followed by tonic (twitching) and clonic (relaxing) muscle contractions. During this time the person might bite his tongue, lose control of body functions, and take very shallow breaths. This usually lasts for two or three minutes and is followed by limpness. When the person regains consciousness he or she may be sleepy, have a headache, be confused, and/or have sore muscles. Most people are able to return to their normal activities after resting. If the seizure begins again, call for emergency assistance.

How to Help Someone During a Seizure

Once started, a seizure cannot be stopped abruptly. Most will end naturally. If you have never seen someone have a seizure, it can be an alarming experience. If you understand what is happening, however, you'll be knowledgeable about what to do.

First, make sure the person is breathing. Loosen clothes around the neck. If the person is having trouble breathing, immediately call for emergency help. Most of the time, a person having a seizure requires no assistance other than caring observation.

If the person appears to be breathing well on his own, take a moment to clear the area of sharp objects or anything else that could be dangerous. If possible, help the person lie on his side. This helps keep their airway open. Protect the patient's head from being bumped if he is having a generalized seizure. **Don't** put anything in the person's mouth.

Most seizures last several minutes. After the seizure ends, allow time for the person to recover. He may be confused for a few moments—this is normal. Help re-orient him. Tell him **who** you are, **where** he is, and **what** happened. Help him find a place to rest until he feels like himself again.

Call for emergency assistance if:
▸ s/he is having difficulty breathing
▸ the person injures him/herself
▸ the seizure lasts more than 10 minutes
▸ a second seizure immediately follows

Treatment

Seizures may be controlled in three ways. The most common is with drugs. The second method is surgery. The third method is a special diet, called a ketogenic diet. Sometimes, a combination of methods is used.

▲ Drugs

Drugs are the most widely used method of controlling seizures. The drugs are prescribed to prevent further seizures or decrease their frequency. They are called *antiepileptic* drugs. Many different antiepileptic drugs are available. The type your doctor prescribes for you depends on the type of seizure you are experiencing.

▲ Surgery

Surgery to remove the tumor may also stop your seizures. If that occurs, the factor that was irritating the brain's electrical system was removed. Or, using sophisticated brain mapping techniques, the neurosurgeon may be able to define the exact area of the brain causing the seizures and surgically remove it.

▲ Ketogenic diet

The ketogenic diet is used to treat epilepsy (recurrent seizures) in children, especially if seizure medications are not effective. The diet is based on a very high intake of fat which causes a chemical imbalance in the body called *ketosis*. Because of the potential side-effects of ketosis, this diet must be prescribed and carefully monitored by a doctor, just as antiepileptic drugs are prescribed and carefully monitored.

About Drug Therapy

There are several important points to remember while you are taking antiepileptic medications.
▸ Antiepileptic drugs work best when there is a steady level of the drug in your body. The drug needs to reach and remain at the ideal level to be effective. Frequent blood tests are required to check the drug levels. Your medications might be adjusted based on the results. Remember to take your medication regularly as prescribed. If you miss a dose, don't double up. Resume your regular schedule and notify your doctor. If you stop taking your medicine abruptly, seizure activity will increase. If you miss more than one dose, or if you notice an increase in your seizures or if you develop a rash, call your doctor for instructions.
▸ There are many medications—both prescription and over-the-counter—that can influence the effectiveness of antiepileptic drugs. Be sure your doctor is aware of *all* the medications you take.

▸ Ask your doctor about operating heavy equipment or having alcoholic drinks.

▸ In the interest of protecting both the public and the driver, all states issue driving guidelines for people who have seizures. To protect yourself, ask your doctor about driving **before you get behind the wheel,** and follow the guidelines.

▸ Do not change the dosage or stop taking your medicine without the approval of your doctor. If one medication doesn't control your seizures, another drug or a combination of drugs may be prescribed.

▸ Most people continue taking antiepileptic medications for several years following their last seizure. Your doctor will outline your treatment plan for you.

Some of the commonly used medications for controlling seizures caused by brain tumors are:

▸ carbamazepine (Tegretol)
▸ gabapentin (Neurontin)
▸ phenobarbital (Luminal)
▸ phenytoin (Dilantin)
▸ divalproex sodium (Depakote)

Several new drugs are available. Your doctor can discuss your medication options with you.

Side-Effects of Drug Therapy

You will be given specific instructions for taking your medication. Your doctor or nurse will tell you the drug's common side-effects, which side-effects you should call the doctor about, and which side-effects should lessen with time.

Because most of the antiepileptic drugs can cause blood or organ disorders, your doctor will perform frequent physical exams and blood tests to avoid these potential effects.

Listed below are the most frequent side-effects of the commonly used antiepileptic drugs. This is not a complete listing, however. Information about

your drug and the circumstances in which to call your doctor should be provided by your healthcare team.

▸ **Carbamazepine (Tegretol)**
Double or blurred vision, dizziness, drowsiness, nausea, headache, skin rash. This drug may decrease the effectiveness of oral contraceptives. Other drugs can cause the blood levels of Tegretol to increase or decrease.

▸ **Gabapentin (Neurontin)**
Dizziness, drowsiness, fatigue, ataxia, sleepiness, nausea, vomiting, slurred speech, skin rash. Should not be taken within two hours of antacids. Neurontin is one of the newer antiepileptic drugs.

▸ **Phenobarbital (Luminal)**
Lack of concentration, sleepiness, hyperactivity, depression, "hangover-like" headache, skin flushing, nausea, vomiting, skin rash. Commonly used for seizures in children. In adults, it may be used with Dilantin, or when other antiepileptic drugs are not effective. Several drugs can increase the effect of phenobarbital.

▸ **Phenytoin (Dilantin)**
Drowsiness, dizziness, low blood pressure, rapid jerky eye movements, clumsy walk, swollen gums, skin rash. Many drugs, prescription (including chemotherapy drugs) and over-the-counter (including aspirins and antacids), can increase or decrease the effectiveness of this drug.

▸ **Valproic acid (Depakene) or divalproex sodium (Depakote)**
Nausea, vomiting, indigestion, diarrhea, abdominal cramps which may lessen with continued use, drowsiness, anorexia or increased appetite, temporary hair loss, photosensitivity. May reduce the effectiveness of oral contraceptives. Do not break or crush the pills as they will irritate the mouth and throat. When used with Dilantin, Depakote may cause Dilantin levels to change.

Notify your doctor immediately if you: have any difficulty breathing, run a temperature, notice the whites of your eyes appear yellow or you have tiny purple spots on your skin, become unusually confused, have difficulty urinating, or bruise easily. Chest pain or inability to arouse someone taking antiepileptic drugs is always a medical emergency.

Managing Common Side-Effects

The following hints may help you manage some common side-effects of antiepileptic drugs.

DROWSINESS OR DIZZINESS

Do not operate equipment or machinery and don't drink alcoholic beverages. Use caution on stairways. Install grab-bars in the shower and next to the toilet (these can be rented from a medical supply store). If the drowsiness persists, contact your doctor.

GUM SWELLING

Good oral hygiene is a vital part of managing this side-effect. If your gums are swollen, try using a mouth care "sponge"— they are available at most drug stores. A soft toothbrush is another option. Avoid mouthwashes containing alcohol as they will further burn and irritate your gums. Look for baking soda-based mouth rinses, or ask your dentist to suggest one. Be sure to tell your dentist about your medication—frequent professional cleanings may help limit gum swelling.

RASH

First, notify your doctor. A rash can indicate an allergic reaction to the drug, or may be due to an increased drug level. If itching accompanies the rash, a cool shower may help—it constricts the blood vessels in the outer layer of your skin. Pat skin dry instead of rubbing. Don't use lotions on the rash unless your doctor or nurse suggests it.

NAUSEA AND VOMITING

Be sure to take your medication with meals to decrease stomach irritation. If stomach upset continues, ask your doctor about antiemetic medication. Antiemetics block the messages to the vomiting center of the brain. Don't use over-the-counter antacids or aspirin-containing preparations for upset stomachs without first checking with your doctor. They may interfere with some antiepileptic drugs.

CONTINUED SEIZURES and IDEAL DRUG LEVELS

Some seizures simply do not respond to a given drug. You may have to try another medication. Be sure to let your doctor know how often you have seizures, and if the side-effects of a particular drug interfere with your quality of life.

Be aware that flu vaccines can increase seizure activity.

CONTINUED SEIZURES and IRREGULAR DRUG LEVELS

Antiepileptics are frequently affected by other medications. If you are experiencing this problem, make a list of all your medications (over-the-counter as well as prescription drugs) and take it to your doctor or pharmacist. Be sure to keep a record of your seizures, particularly the frequency and type. Discuss this with your doctor, and ask about other options for controlling your seizures.

For more information about seizures and seizure medications, contact the Epilepsy Foundation of America ▾ 4351 Garden City Drive ▾ Landover, MD 20785 ▾ (800) 332-1000 ▾ Fax (301) 577-2684 ▾ E-mail postmaster@efa.org ▾ Web site http://www.efa.org. There is a small charge for some of their publications.

Chapter 14

Brain Tumors in Children

Children with brain tumors have symptoms and needs that differ considerably from their adult counterparts. Their developing bodies and brains require special care and consideration. Throughout their treatment and years of follow-up, their caregivers should include specialists from several disciplines, such as neurologists, endocrinologists, ophthalmologists, psychologists, and possibly other specialists.

The most common childhood brain tumors are different from the most common adult brain tumors in that:
- their most frequent locations are different
- they often behave differently than similar tumors in adults, and many have a better prognosis
- they are often treated differently from those in adults, particularly in very young children

Children who have brain tumors require special care because their bodies and brains are still developing. The young patient who receives state-of-the-art treatment from an experienced, multi-disciplinary pediatric healthcare team often has a better chance of survival and quality of life than their adult counterparts.

We hope the discussion and suggestions in this chapter help you manage the unique challenges you face as the parent of a child with a brain tumor.

See Chapter 7, *Types of Brain and Spinal Cord Tumors* for more detailed descriptions of these tumors.

Background

With only about 2,200 children diagnosed with a brain tumor in the United States each year, it is a rare disease of childhood. The most common presenting symptoms are a history of flu-like symptoms; frequent headaches that are worse in the morning and are associated with nausea or vomiting; a wobbly walk; a decline in school performance; and changes in vision. Symptoms that don't improve after a reasonable period of time should be investigated.

More brain tumors are found in children age 7 and younger than in older children, and they tend to be more common in boys than girls.

The good news is that today's sophisticated technology allows for improved diagnosis and treatment. Much has been learned about childhood brain tumors over the past ten years, and survival rates have improved dramatically for specific tumor types. Pediatric treatment teams that specialize in childhood brain tumors offer a multi-disciplinary approach to treatment. Many children return to their previous lifestyles although many years of specialized rehabilitative treatment may be necessary—due to disabilities caused by the treatment required to combat the tumor, and difficulties caused by the tumor itself. In addition, special education services may be necessary.

A particular challenge for the very young child with a brain tumor is the extremely long treatment plan. In many cases, chemotherapy treatment, while not curative, will be used to delay the more definitive radiation treatments. Studies indicate that far less damage occurs to the young developing brain if radiation is delayed until the child is at least three years of age, or preferably

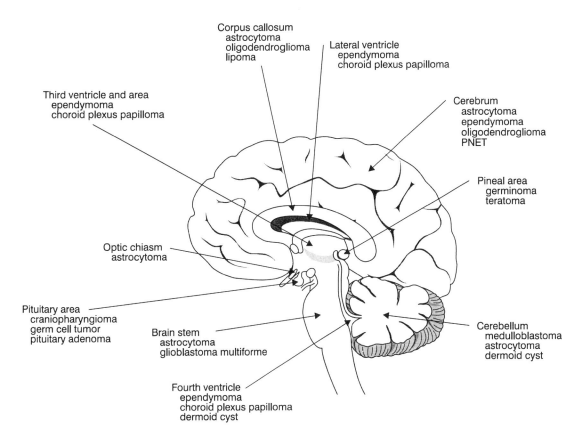

Location of Common Childhood Brain Tumors

older. Therefore, depending on the age of the child at onset, a child may spend many years cycling on and off treatment as the treatment team develops the optimal plan.

Common Childhood Tumors

Childhood brain tumors are classified by their biological characteristics and their location in the brain. About half of all pediatric brain tumors are **infratentorial**—they occur in the structures below the tentorium. This area, also called the **posterior fossa**, contains the fourth ventricle, the brain stem and the cerebellum.

▲ Common infratentorial tumors

BRAIN STEM GLIOMA _____
Tumors of any grade can occur in this area. They represent 10-20% of all pediatric brain tumors. About 60-80% of brain stem gliomas are diffuse and require treatment with radiation and some-

times other forms of treatment as well. Smaller, more localized lesions, can at times be treated with surgery or chemotherapy with or without radiotherapy. Chemotherapy to delay radiation is given to children under age 3. Clinical trials using chemotherapy and radiation therapy are available (see *Glioma, Brain Stem* in Chapter 7).

CEREBELLAR ASTROCYTOMA _____
This is usually a low-grade tumor which rarely spreads. Following surgery, no further treatment might be given if the tumor is completely removed. Cerebellar astrocytomas represent about 15% of pediatric brain tumors (see *Astrocytoma* in Chapter 7).

EPENDYMOMA _____
(*Separate publication available. See page 137*)
Infratentorial ependymomas represent about 7% of childhood brain tumors. It may spread throughout the entire central nervous system, but is usually localized. Total surgical removal improves the

likelihood of disease control. Surgery followed by radiation therapy is the standard treatment, although chemotherapy may be used with radiation therapy for partially resected tumors or may be given to delay radiation for children under age 3. Clinical trials using chemotherapy are available (see *Ependymoma* in Chapter 7).

MEDULLOBLASTOMA

(Separate publication available. See page 137)
A fast growing tumor located in the cerebellum of children and young adults, it tends to spread throughout the central nervous system via the cerebrospinal fluid. Fifteen to twenty percent of childhood brain tumors are medulloblastomas.

In children three years of age or older, standard treatment consists of surgery followed by radiation therapy, usually with chemotherapy. Further treatment is based on risk evaluation.

Standard-risk patients have no residual tumor after surgery and no metastases. *High-risk* patients have residual tumor after surgery, evidence of metastasis, or possible brain stem involvement. For children younger than 3 years of age, chemotherapy is usually given to delay radiation therapy. For some children, chemotherapy may be the only additional treatment needed.

Many clinical trials are available for this common pediatric brain tumor (see *Medulloblastoma* in Chapter 7).

▲ Common supratentorial tumors

ASTROCYTOMA

Astrocytomas of all grades may occur. If the tumor is a low-grade astrocytoma located within the cerebral hemispheres, no treatment beyond surgery may be necessary. Radiation and chemotherapy are often given following surgery for higher-grade tumors for children over the age of 3. Chemotherapy may be used to delay radiation in children younger than 3. Clinical trials using chemotherapy are available (see *Astrocytoma* in Chapter 7).

EPENDYMOMA

(Separate publication available. See page 137)
Standard treatment is surgery followed by radiation therapy for children over the age of 3. Chemotherapy to delay radiation is often used in children younger than 3. Clinical trials using chemotherapy are available (see *Ependymoma* in Chapter 7).

CRANIOPHARYNGIOMA

This benign tumor, located near the pituitary gland, represents about 5-13% of pediatric brain tumors. A craniopharyngioma causes problems by compression rather than invasion. Treatment may be surgery or radiation therapy or both (see *Craniopharyngioma* in Chapter 7).

GERM CELL TUMOR

Usually located near the pineal gland, this tumor may spread throughout the central nervous system. The usual treatment is radiation therapy, often with chemotherapy for children over the age of 3. Chemotherapy to delay radiation may be used with children younger than 3. Clinical trials using chemotherapy are available (see *Germ Cell Tumors* in Chapter 7).

OPTIC TRACT GLIOMA

This is usually a slow-growing astrocytoma. They represent about 4% of childhood brain tumors.

Depending on the location and extent of the tumor, treatment may consist of "wait and see," radiation therapy, chemotherapy or surgery. Chemotherapy may be used to delay radiation in children younger than 3 (see *Glioma, Optic* in Chapter 7).

PINEAL TUMOR

Several different types of tumors may be found in the pineal gland or pineal area. Treatment depends on the specific tumor, its location and its tendency to spread. Most tumors should be biopsied, although at times diagnosis can be made by analysis of the cerebrospinal fluid for tumor markers. Treatment after surgery is usually radiation therapy. Chemotherapy is often used, especially for mixed-germ cells or to delay radiation until age 3 (see *Pineal Tumors* and *Pineal Region Tumors* in Chapter 7).

PNET

This fast growing tumor can spread throughout the central nervous system. Standard therapy is surgery followed by radiation therapy, usually with chemotherapy for children over the age of 3. Chemotherapy to delay radiation may be used in children younger than 3. Clinical trials using chemotherapy are available (see *PNET* in Chapter 7).

Treatment Considerations

Surgery, often followed by radiotherapy and/or chemotherapy is the standard treatment for most pediatric brain tumors. Low-grade gliomas and other benign tumors may be treated with surgery alone, if most of the tumor can be removed. Some brain stem gliomas, optic tract gliomas, and germ cell tumors might be treated without surgical confirmation. Chemotherapy has been increasingly used for childhood brain tumors, especially in medulloblastoma and chiasmatic gliomas.

Because of the potential for serious side-effects on the developing brain, radiotherapy is usually delayed in children under the age of 3. Surgery and/or chemotherapy is preferred until the child is older. After the age of 3, a second surgery or radiotherapy is given if the tumor progresses.

The Pediatric Oncology Group (POG) and the Children's Cancer Study Group (CCG) are clinical cooperative groups funded by the National Cancer Institute (NCI). Both groups offer clinical trials for pediatric brain tumor patients. In addition, many other institutions conduct clinical trials. Lists of medical centers and physicians participating in clinical trials are available from NCI's Cancer Information Service at 1-800-4-CANCER. Or, call our office at 1-800-886-2282 for a listing of physicians who offer investigative treatments for pediatric brain tumor patients.

Because brain tumors in children are uncommon, medical centers participating in clinical trials usually offer the most up-to-date treatment options. The skills of various pediatric neuro-specialists are often necessary, and are commonly available at those medical centers.

Treatment Side-Effects

Some treatment methods, while increasing survival, may have significant long-term side-effects on young children. Depending on the type of treatment, side-effects may include a change in overall intelligence, learning disabilities, attitudinal problems, fatigue, depression and changes in personality. These symptoms are especially common after whole-brain radiation therapy. Hormonal problems are also common. Prior to treatment, your child may undergo neuropsychological testing. The results are used as a baseline for future evaluation. Testing for school problems should be used to devise more appropriate and tailored school programs.

Long Term Follow-Up

Children are followed for many years after treatment to monitor the effectiveness of their treatment and to check for potential long-term side-effects.

Scans are repeated about twice a year for the first two years following treatment for a low-grade tumor, then about once a year until the child is older. If the tumor was high-grade, scanning is done every 3 months for the first two years, then less frequently when the child is older. Endocrine evaluations and neuropsychological testing are also routinely performed, usually on a yearly basis.

Potential complications to be aware of, especially following radiation therapy or combination chemotherapy and radiation therapy, include:

» decreased levels of growth hormone
» decreased levels of thyroid hormone

» delayed spinal growth (from radiation to the spine)

» decreased intellect or learning disabilities, particularly if the child was very young when radiated

Replacement therapy can be initiated to overcome the hormone deficiencies; rehabilitation and special education can enhance the quality of life for other treatment effects. Children with brain tumors often have several disabling conditions (from tumor and/or treatment) which need to be addressed, such as visual impairments, hearing loss, physical disabilities and cognitive delays. In addition, residual tumor, hydrocephalus, seizure activity and tumor necrosis can continue to affect the child long after treatment has been discontinued. It can be particularly difficult for parents to find information that addresses the inter-relationship of all these factors and how to best manage their child's overall care. Parents often act as the case manager for their child, advocating in educational and medical settings to find the best services.

Untreated children have little chance of survival. The risk of incurring long-term treatment side-effects must be weighed against the outcome if a child is not treated.

Recurrences

The majority of recurrences in children occur within three to five years of initial treatment. Recurrences five to ten years after treatment do occur, but are uncommon in the more malignant tumors.

Talking With Your Child

This section applies to the children who are patients as well as their siblings—young brothers and sisters need to be treated as carefully as the child with the brain tumor.

Most young children are unaware of the changes their disease might have on their future. They are often acutely conscious of the seriousness of their illness yet might not be able to express their concerns to you.

Very young children are often most concerned about being separated from their parents during treatment. They need reassurance that they will be cared for, and that their parents will return. They need to know honestly when something is going to hurt. Give your child a way to handle pain—have him squeeze your hand, or suggest he count to three and blow. These techniques can help divert his attention and relieve some of the anxiety when the procedure is done the next time. Reward your child: hugs go a long way in relieving the pain of a needlestick.

Young children should be told only as much as they can understand. Take your cues from their questions. Answer simply and honestly, but offer only the information they ask for.

Older children can be given choices in their treatment—which arm should be poked today, or whether the blood test comes before or after a shower. Choices help children have some control over what is happening to them. They need to have their fears addressed directly; children have a limited knowledge of their disease and their imaginations may run wild. Honesty is vital.

Provide the opportunity for your child to express his fears, sadness and concerns. "Would you like to talk about this?" can be difficult for you to ask, but might be just the opening your child needs. Keeping a diary or audio-taping a journal of their illness might help a child express some of his anxieties. Our booklet, *Alex's Journey,* is the story of a child with a brain tumor. Written for ages 9-13, it helps children understand their disease and lets them know they are not alone. To obtain a copy, see page 137.

A brain tumor poses a frustrating obstacle for the teenager attempting to achieve independence. The illness necessitates dependence on family and medical personnel just at the time the teen is ready to take his own place in society. Educational plans might be delayed. Keeping and making new friends may be difficult because of physical changes in his appearance. Support groups consisting of other teens experiencing the same disease might help him to form friendships.

Remember to include your child's teacher in your plans. Lessons can be modified or completed at home. An informed teacher can keep the class apprised of your child's progress, and prepare the class for his or her return. For more information, see our publication *When Your Child Returns to School* (see page 137).

Most pediatric treatment centers offer child life specialists, art therapists or social workers who can help you, and your family, through this time. Seek out the resources available to you. For example, you might be interested in oncology or disability-related camps for your children, or local support groups for siblings of chronically ill or disabled children. Your treatment center social worker should be able to help you locate these groups. Or, call us for assistance if you need help in locating the resources you need.

Disability-Related Resources

PARENT TRAINING CENTERS
Each state has at least one center that serves parents of children with special needs. To obtain the number for your state's resource center, call TAPP at (617) 236-7210.

Parent training centers are funded by each state's Department of Education. They usually work closely with the Department of Rehabilitative Services. Their offices are commonly staffed by parents of children with special needs who can help with questions about a wide range of topics.

NICHCY (National Information Center for Children and Youth with Disabilities)
(800) 695-0285 ▲ http://www.nichcy.org
This national information and referral center provides information on specific disabilities, interventions, special education, educational rights, transitional services and family concerns.

HEATH RESOURCE CENTER (National Clearinghouse on Post-Secondary Education for Individuals with Disabilities)
1 DuPont Circle, NW, Suite 800, Washington, DC 20036 ▲ (202) 939-9320 ▲
E-mail Heath@ace.nche.edu ▲
http://www.acenet.edu/programs/Heath
A program of the American Council on Education, HEATH provides information about support services, accommodations, policies and procedures at American campuses, vocational-technical schools and other post-secondary education facilities.

CHILDHOOD CANCER OMBUDSMAN PROGRAM
(301) 515-2900
A project of The Childhood Brain Tumor Foundation, this program helps families access adequate health care coverage; educational, vocational and rehabilitative services; employment and insurance discrimination information.

THE CANDLELIGHTERS CHILDHOOD CANCER FOUNDATION
(800) 366-2223 ▲ http://www.candlelighters.org
Publishes a free booklet *Educating the Child with Cancer* which includes a chapter specific to children with brain tumors and chapters on siblings, school re-entry programs, legal rights of children in special education and further resources.

Roger Packer, MD, Colleen Snyder and Elizabeth Irvin of The Childhood Brain Tumor Foundation contributed to this chapter. We are very grateful for their assistance.
The Childhood Brain Tumor Foundation ▲ 20312 Watkins Meadow Drive ▲ Germantown, MD 20876 ▲ (301) 515-2900

Chapter 15

Comfort and Coping

You might still be trying to make sense out of the words *brain tumor*. You and those near to you are frightened and probably feeling isolated. Comfort and control seem like a dream.

This chapter offers suggestions and advice from professionals who specialize in helping people cope, and from other patients and those close to them who have had experiences similar to yours. We hope some of their ideas work for you.

Understanding Your Disease

For many people, understanding is the foundation for coping. Arm yourself with information.

Listen carefully to your doctors and nurses when they explain your illness and treatment options. They are the best source of information about *your* brain tumor. Don't be afraid to ask questions. Most healthcare professionals want patients to be knowledgeable so they can be active members of their treatment team.

You probably have lots of questions. List them in a notebook, placing the most important questions at the top of the list. Bring your questions to your doctor and jot down the answers. It can be helpful to have someone with you. A relative or friend can provide moral support and also help you remember what was said. If it's okay with your doctor, bring a tape recorder with you. You will then be able to listen to the doctor again in the comfort of your own home.

During your doctors' visits, ask for written information about your brain tumor, your symptoms, suggested treatments, and your medications. Before you leave the doctor's office, make sure you understand any instructions you were given. For example, do you have another appointment? If so, when is it? If you are scheduled to have additional tests, do you know when and where to go? Ask the nurse to write important dates and instructions in your notebook.

Telling Family and Friends

Many people find that it helps to share their news with others.

Telling your family you have a brain tumor isn't easy. If you are uncomfortable telling them, consider having a family conference with your doctor. When you speak with your family, remember that written information about brain tumors is available and can help explain your situation more easily. Like you, your family needs time to understand the diagnosis. If your family understands your illness and the options available to you, they will likely be tremendously supportive and helpful.

Social workers can help you find ways to share your feelings with your family, and help you and your family cope. Most hospitals have social work departments. You can also find social workers at community centers, government health agencies and schools.

If you are a parent with young children and you have a brain tumor, try to anticipate your children's concerns. Children use their imaginations to fill in the gaps and their fantasies can cause undue fears and anxieties. Give children information in words they understand. Use their questions as a guide to the amount of information they want. Be prepared for questions that aren't easily answered; reply honestly and simply. Young people often have remarkable insight and can be a source of great comfort.

There are many books available that can help parents explain their illness to children. Although most of these books are about cancer, the advice

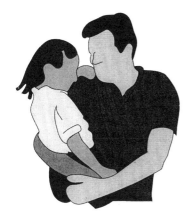

they contain is useful for many illnesses. Read these books with your children; offer them the opportunity to ask questions and to express their fears and concerns.

Most importantly, remember that children of all ages need to be reassured that you have planned for their needs. Explain those plans and arrangements to your children, making sure they know you are still very much involved, even if from a distance.

If friends offer to help, accept their offers. You benefit from the help, and your friends feel needed. Groceries, laundry, a meal on the day of your doctor visit, transportation to the clinic for therapy—there are many possibilities. Keep a "Wish List" of things you "wish" you had the time to do. When someone offers to help, reach for that list.

Although most people will be supportive, some will be unable to deal with or even acknowledge your illness. Also, be prepared for well-meaning neighbors who insist upon telling you stories about "miraculous" cures. Thank them for their concern, but remember to put their tales in perspective. There are many different types of brain tumors, and many different treatments. What

works for one person may not be appropriate for another. Ask your doctor.

Second Opinions

Not everyone wants, or needs, a second opinion. But maybe you'd like to speak to another doctor about your diagnosis or possible treatments. Or perhaps your insurance company requires a second opinion before they authorize payment for a treatment. It is very important, however, to make sure it is safe to delay treatment long enough to obtain a second opinion.

If you decide to seek another opinion, there are several different ways to go about it. Your doctor can suggest another specialist, and might even make the appointment for you. Hospital-based physician referral services can provide you with the names of doctors who practice at their facilities. Professional organizations, insurance companies, or your family doctor might be referral sources. Or, you may already know of another doctor you want to consult.

If speaking to another doctor would lessen your anxiety, then do it. Second opinions are considered standard medical practice. A consultation might increase your understanding about your disease and your options for treatment. It is important to choose a doctor you can communicate with, one you feel comfortable working with, and one who offers the treatment options you're interested in.

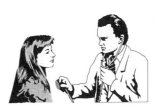

After deciding with whom you want to consult, call and ask how to go about getting a second opinion, and what fees, if any, might be involved. Many doctors will agree to consult by telephone. Others require you to make an appointment. Either way, if the doctor agrees to consult with you, he'll need your medical records. Ask for a list of the records that are needed, and arrange for them to be sent. After the records have been received, and if the doctor has agreed to consult by telephone, ask when to expect the call.

Obtaining Your Medical Records

The laws for obtaining your medical records vary by state. Many states allow records to be released directly to the patient upon request. Other states require that medical records be sent directly to the consulting physician.

The quickest way to obtain those records is from your doctor's office. Pathology, surgical and consultation reports as well as records of office visits are generally kept with the chart in your doctor's office. Written reports from scans are also kept in the chart (but probably not the scans themselves). The office may charge you for copying the records, and they can forward them directly to the consulting doctor's office.

If your doctor does not have your scans, call the Radiology Department of the hospital where the scans were done. Request copies of any scans, x-rays or myelograms that you need. **Never send an original through the mail**. Copies of scans can be expensive, and there may be many of them, so it's a good idea to determine exactly which ones you will need for the consultation.

Pathology slides are usually stored in the Pathology Department of the hospital where the surgery was performed. Some slides can be copied. To obtain your slides, call the hospital's Pathology Department. Again, there may be a charge to duplicate the slides.

Written reports of your hospitalization are kept in the Medical Records Department of the hospital. Call that department and ask how to obtain your records. Some hospitals require a written authorization from the patient to release the records. Again, there may be a charge for copying the records.

Find out if the records will be released to you or sent to the consulting doctor. If you are to pick up the records, ask where and when they will be available. If the records are to be forwarded, find out when they will be sent and by what method. Call the consulting doctor's office to verify that they have been received.

Your Feelings

When you first heard your diagnosis, you were probably shocked. Chances are you understood very little of what you were told at that time. Those were perfectly normal reactions. Most people experience some or all of the following feelings following the diagnosis of a brain tumor.

Denial—disbelief or lack of concern over the diagnosis—is normal for some. It may take time to accept the news. Some may initially pretend it hasn't happened. Others may be in a state of shock. "How could I have a brain tumor?" or "Why me?" are common questions. Some people may refuse to discuss or even acknowledge their diagnosis.

Guilt—when something overwhelming happens, people try to blame someone. When you blame yourself, you feel guilt. People ask: Is this a punishment? Did I do something to deserve this? The cause of most brain tumors is unknown. Nothing you did, said or thought made this happen.

Anger—at your husband, wife, children, neighbor, boss, doctor or anyone and everyone—is not unusual. You may say hurting, bitter things you don't really mean and later regret. Small children may kick or bite to show their anger. Hidden anger sometimes causes irritability, sleeplessness, fatigue, over-eating, or over-drinking.

Depression—or grief at the loss of your previous lifestyle may occur. While physical activity may be the last thing you feel you have the energy for at this time, it often helps the most.

Later, or when you complete treatment and your life becomes less hectic, the enormity of all that is happening becomes vivid. Now, you need to cope with your fears and anxiety.

It is normal for people to experience anxiety when going through stressful times. Many people feel "anxious" while waiting for test results or when returning to the doctor for follow-up visits. Symptoms of anxiety include a sense of fear, a feeling that "something bad" is going to happen, a rapid heart rate, perspiration, nausea, shortness of breath, dizziness, or a feeling of unreality.

It is important to talk to your doctor about your physical symptoms even though they may be psychologically based. If your doctor determines that the symptoms are the result of anxiety, he may suggest medication or a visit with a psychiatrist, psychologist or social worker. Sometimes, just the reassurance that your doctor provides will be enough to relieve your anxiety.

While many of the feelings people experience are normal and can be worked through, there are some for whom these changes are overwhelming. Those people may become very depressed, and need help in dealing with those feelings. Some of the symptoms of major depression are: persistent depression or no feelings whatsoever; irritability; loss of enjoyment and pleasure in people or activities that are normally enjoyable; difficulty sleeping—such as trouble falling asleep or waking too early and being unable to fall asleep again; loss of appetite; or wanting to give up or to inflict self-harm. When these feelings persist for more than a few weeks, or when they are severe, it is important to bring the symptoms to the attention of a doctor. The doctor will determine whether these are signs of major depression and if so will provide direction. The doctor may prescribe medication or suggest a psychiatric consultation. Depression is treatable, but first it must be diagnosed.

There is no magic pattern for dealing with your emotions. One day you may feel better, and the next day feel upset again. Not everyone shows their emotions, nor does everyone have the same kinds of feelings. If this is your first experience with crisis, you will learn which coping methods work best for you. Hopefully, those who deal with their emotions in an unpressured way will begin to accept the reshaping of their lives, facing it with a realistic amount of hope and a determined attitude.

Living Your Life

Part of our identity is how we present ourselves to others. An undesired change in the way we look upsets us and those around us.

Hair lost during surgery, radiation, or chemotherapy often grows back, but may take months. Wigs are available for both men and women. If you find a wig uncomfortable, consider 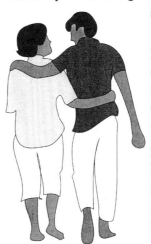 a scarf or a loose hat.

Look through your closet for the clothes you look best in. Or, treat yourself to a new blouse or tie. When you look good, you feel better. Many hospitals offer make-up and hair sessions for those who have gone through cancer treatments. The workshops give you tips about your appearance, and are great for your self-confidence.

Many people with a brain tumor have questions about sex. Can I still have sex? How soon after surgery can I have sex? Will my treatments affect my desire for sex? Talk to a member of your healthcare team—they can answer your questions and provide suggestions.

Your desire for sex may decrease temporarily because you're tired, you feel unattractive, or you fear hurting yourself. Or your partner may be afraid of hurting you. For the time being, consider replacing sexual activity with non-sexual physical closeness such as holding hands, kissing or hugging. Find activities you can comfortably share and special times to be alone.

You may feel tired due to medications, treatments, and traveling to and from your treatments. Be realistic—keeping up with your usual responsibilities may be difficult. Set priorities. Do only what has to be done, and if you still have the energy or inclination, then consider other chores or errands. Call upon friends and neighbors to help. Plan frequent rest periods during the day. Save your energy for special events or unavoidable chores.

Make time to be good to yourself. Take up a hobby or learn a new craft. Visit your beautician or barber. Go to the library and check out those books you always wanted to read. Keep a diary. Look for ways to enjoy yourself.

Coping with Stress

For most people, a fear of the unknown and an uncertain future cause great stress. This is normal. Give yourself permission to be temporarily overwhelmed. Then, take a deep breath and begin to think about the things you can control.

Ask family and friends to help with household responsibilities. Get someone to complete medical forms and claims. Participate in planning your treatment. Help determine your medication or treatment schedules. Decide which chores are important, and which can be temporarily ignored. Choose to share your experience with others, or not. The choice is yours.

Reducing stress means being kind to yourself. Soft classical music, attending a ball game, a mid-afternoon nap—all are relaxing activities that also pamper you.

If you are a family member or friend, you need to permit yourself some "time off" to take care of your own needs, despite the confusion of the situation. Call upon other relatives or friends to serve as relief workers so you can take much needed breaks.

Communication is an important part of reducing stress. Talk to your family about your needs, feelings, and responsibilities. Listen to their concerns, as well. Sometimes one person will take on too many responsibilities. Or, in trying to protect others, a family member may not express her/his own needs. Taking the time to talk—about what needs to be done and who can reasonably do it—allows everyone to feel useful and avoids feelings of resentment. Relaxation, meditation or imagery techniques can also help reduce stress for you and your family. Consider taking a class together.

Birthdays, holidays, or anniversaries can be a difficult time for your family. Anxiousness or irritability around these days is normal. Plan ahead and make activities simple and memorable.

Close friends, religious leaders, or your family physician can be a source of emotional and physical strength. Friends may be able to search for community and medical resources of value to you. Contact your library, local civic organizations, village hall, or religious institutions. Many community programs are available—learn what they are and take advantage of their services. Each resource you find makes it easier for you and your family to cope with your new situation.

Finding A Support Group

Most of us don't want to be alone when facing a crisis. Emotional support from family, friends, and

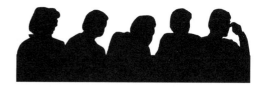

loved ones gives us comfort and strength, but may not be enough. There is often a need to connect with someone in the same situation.

Patients and families often find help through brain tumor support groups. A support group is a gathering of people seeking to share their experiences. They come for emotional, and possibly, spiritual support. Within the safety of a support group, many people are able to share their fears and concerns about day-to-day problems and the future.

There are different types of support groups— for adults, for parents of children with brain tumors, for children and siblings. Most of these groups also welcome concerned friends. If you are not comfortable with a particular group or it doesn't meet your needs, try another one.

Selected Resources For Support Services

▲ American Brain Tumor Association

▸ (800) 886-2282 ▲ http://www.abta.org
Our "comfort and coping" services will provide you with personalized, timely information and assistance. Support groups, a pen-pal program, social service consultations, housing and transportation information during treatment, and much more, are yours for the asking. All services are free of charge to patients and their families.

▲ American Cancer Society

▸ (800) ACS-2345 ▲ http://www.cancer.org
A nation-wide, community-based organization which focuses on research and education. Some chapters offer patient services such as transport-ation assistance, housing, financial aid and wig lending banks. Their toll-free information line refers callers to local ACS offices.

▲ Cancer Care, Inc.

▸ (800) 813-HOPE ▲ http://www.cancercare.org
Their toll-free counseling line provides counseling, information, referrals and assistance to cancer patients, their families and loved ones.

▲ Candlelighters Childhood Cancer Foundation

▸ (800) 366-2223 ▲ http://www.candlelighters.org
Exists to educate, support and advocate for families of children with cancer, survivors of childhood cancer and the professionals who care for them. They offer a network of peer-support groups for parents, a Youth Newsletter, a biblio-graphy of cancer related materials, an Ombudsman Program for insurance concerns and bereavement counseling.

▲ Coping® Magazine

▸ (615) 790-2400
A bi-monthly national magazine for cancer patients, families and oncology professionals. A sample issue is available upon request at no charge. Subscriptions are $18.00 per year.

▲ National Coalition for Cancer Survivorship

▸ (888) 650-9127 ▲ http://www.cansearch.org
Acts as a clearinghouse and helps cancer survivors, their families and friends find local support groups, learn health insurance options and prevent employment bias.

▲ National Family Caregivers Association

▸ (800) 896-3650 ▲ http://www.nfcacares.org
Provides education, support, respite care and advocacy for caregivers. Their toll-free information line provides referrals to caregiver support groups as well as information on how to start a caregivers support group.

▲ National Hospice Organization

▸ (800) 658-8898 ▲ http://www.nho.org
Promotes quality care for the terminally ill and their families. Their help line refers callers to local hospices and they can also inform callers whether a facility is licensed and Medicare certified.

Chapter 16

Questions to Ask Your Healthcare Team

Whether you are just beginning treatment, are a long term survivor, or somewhere in between, you probably have some unasked or unanswered questions. You might be concerned about your symptoms or want to ask about treatment options. You may have obtained copies of your medical records and read something you don't understand. Or perhaps you have concerns about your routine activities. We encourage you to ask questions of your healthcare team. Your doctors and nurses are familiar with your health, and can respond with personalized answers which cannot—*and often should not*—be answered by outside sources.

By asking questions you're participating in your healthcare. By gathering information, you'll feel more comfortable making decisions about your treatment plan.

Make a list of your questions and bring them with you when you visit your doctor. **Be sure the questions that concern you the most are at the top of the list**. If you think of other questions after you return home, begin a list for the next visit.

If you want to bring family or friends with you when you visit your doctor, make an appointment for a conference. Let the receptionist know the purpose of your visit—that way, an adequate block of time can be set aside.

In this chapter, we offer some sample questions you may want to ask at various times during your illness. You probably will modify this list based on your particular concerns and situation.

Your First Visit

Many people don't remember much when their doctor first tells them they have a serious disease. Try to come away with some basic information.

- Where is the tumor located?
- Based on the scans, do you have an idea of the type of tumor?
- What is the next step? Do I need more tests? Do I need to see any specialists?
- Until we know more, should I continue my daily routine? Can I work? Should I drive?
- Do I need to take any medication? If so, what is it for? What are the side-effects?

About Insurance

After your first visit, you need to verify your healthcare insurance coverage. The answers to most of your insurance questions can be found in the insurance policy itself or the policy manual. If you don't have a copy, now is the time to obtain one.

For **employer-provided health insurance**, contact your employer's Human Resources office or your benefits manager and ask for the manual. For **individual policies**, call your insurance agent. For **Medicare/Medicaid** coverage, call the Medicare Hotline at (800) 638-6833. For **CHIP** coverage (Comprehensive Health Insurance Programs) through your state, call your state Department of Insurance. If you are not insured, call the social workers at the hospital where you will be treated. They can help find resources to assist you.

Be sure you know the answers to these questions:
- Do you need to obtain pre-certification for hospitalization or treatment? If so, who do you call? (When you call, be sure to record the name of the person you are speaking with and the "case number" assigned to your claim.)
- Do you need to obtain a second opinion before non-emergency surgery? If so, are there any stipulations as to who provides the second opinion?
- Do you need to stay within a particular network of hospitals or physicians to receive your benefits? Do you have a current list of those providers? What will happen if you are treated "outside the network?"
- Will your insurance cover investigational treatment if you choose it?

Seeing a Specialist

One of your next visits will likely be to a specialist to discuss your treatment. Regardless of whether the next step is surgery, radiation, chemotherapy or another form of treatment, the basic questions are very much the same. You'll want to know:
- What treatment is being recommended?
- What is the goal of this treatment?
- What are the potential benefits of this treatment?
- What will happen if I don't have this treatment or if I postpone it?
- Are there other options besides this treatment?
- Is this an experimental treatment?
- What are the risks and side-effects of this treatment?
- Will I need any more tests before this treatment begins?
- How will we know if this treatment was effective?
- What type of follow-up will I need?

Following Treatment

Now is the time to begin re-defining "normal" in your life. It's a time to slow down and be good to yourself. When you finish your last treatment, be sure you know:
- When is my next doctor visit? Which doctor do I see?
- When is my next scan?
- Do I need any medications? If so, are there any potential side-effects?
- Can I work?
- Can I drive?
- Can I exercise and if so, do I have any limitations?
- What type of diet should I follow?

Living With a Brain Tumor

As time goes by, you and your family may have questions about issues common to all people living with a brain tumor—patients and family members alike. Those issues may involve:
- financial concerns
- employment issues
- obtaining new health insurance
- sexuality
- forming new relationships
- starting or adding to your family
- parenting
- counseling or support groups
- rehabilitative services
- cosmetic and image interests

As more brain tumor patients become survivors, there are increasing resources for answers to these concerns. Call our social worker at (800) 886-2282 if you need help in finding those resources.

Brain Tumor Classification

A single, universal system for classifying brain and spinal cord tumors is desirable so that: 1) the same diagnosis is made by all neuro-pathologists who examine a particular tumor; 2) there is a rationale for recommending a specific treatment; and 3) there is a uniform basis for evaluating the effectiveness of various therapies.

Most institutions follow the new World Health Organization (WHO) classification system, which is based on the tumor's cell of origin and its biological behavior:

- how fast it is growing
- if it is local or spreading
- whether it is exceeding its food and oxygen supply, causing a center core of dead tumor cells
- how abnormal its appearance is

In the WHO system, tumors are graded I to IV—grade I tumors are slow growing and relatively normal appearing under the microscope, grade IV tumors are rapid growing malignancies. A three-tier system (which groups tumors into low, mid and high-grades), and a five-tier system (benign tumors are grade I and malignant, aggressive tumors are grade V) also exist and are used at some institutions. It is important for you to know which classification system was used to identify your tumor.

This *Primer of Brain Tumors* uses the new World Health Organization (WHO) classification of brain tumors system*, which is listed below.

1 **Neuroepithelial Tumors**
   a.   *Astrocytic Tumors*
      1)   Astrocytomas
            Variants: Fibrillary
                     Protoplasmic
                     Gemistocytic
      2)   Anaplastic Astrocytoma
      3)   Glioblastoma Multiforme
            Variants: Giant cell glioblastoma
                     Gliosarcoma
      4)   Pilocytic Astrocytoma
      5)   Pleomorphic xanthoastrocytoma
      6)   Subependymal giant cell astrocytoma
                (Tuberous sclerosis)

   b.   *Oligodendroglial Tumors*
      1)   Oligodendroglioma
      2)   Anaplastic (malignant) oligodendroglioma

   c.   *Ependymal Tumors*
      1)   Ependymoma
            Variants: Cellular
                     Papillary
                     Clear cell
      2)   Anaplastic (malignant) ependymoma
      3)   Myxopapillary ependymoma
      4)   Subependymoma

   d.   *Mixed Gliomas*
      1)   Oligo-astrocytoma
      2)   Anaplastic (malignant) oligo-astrocytoma
      3)   Others (*e.g.* ependymo-astrocytoma)

   e.   *Choroid Plexus Tumors*
      1)   Choroid plexus papilloma
      2)   Choroid plexus carcinoma

f. *Neuroepithelial Tumors of Uncertain Origin*
1) Astroblastoma
2) Polar spongioblastoma
3) Gliomatosis cerebri

g. *Neuronal and Mixed Neuronal-glial Tumors*
1) Gangliocytoma
2) Dysplastic gangliocytoma of cerebellum (Lhermitte-Duclos)
3) Desmoplastic infantile ganglioglioma (DIG)
4) Dysembryoplastic neuroepithelial tumor (DNT)
5) Ganglioglioma
6) Anaplastic (malignant) ganglioglioma
7) Central neurocytoma
8) Paraganglioma of the filum terminale
9) Olfactory neuroblastoma (esthesioneuroblastoma)
   Variant: Olfactory neuroepithelioma

h. *Pineal Parenchyma Tumors*
1) Pineocytoma
2) Pineoblastoma
3) Mixed / transitional pineal tumors

i. *Embryonal Tumors*
1) Medulloepithelioma
2) Neuroblastoma
   Variant: Ganglioneuroblastoma
3) Ependymoblastoma
4) Primitive neuroectodermal tumors (PNETs)
5) Medulloblastoma
   Variants: Desmoplastic medulloblastoma
             Medullomyoblastoma
             Melanotic medulloblastoma

2 Cranial and Spinal Nerve Tumors

a. *Schwannoma (neurilemmoma, neurinoma)*
   Variants: Cellular
             Plexiform
             Melanotic

b. *Neurofibroma*
1) Circumscribed (solitary)
2) Plexiform

c. *Malignant Peripheral Nerve Sheath tumor (MPNST) (Neurogenic sarcoma, Anaplastic neurofibroma, "Malignant schwannoma")*

Variants: Epithelioid MPNST with divergent mesenchymal and/or epithelial differentiation
Melanotic

3 Meningeal Tumors

a. *Meningothelial Cell Tumors*
1) Meningioma
   Variants: Meningothelial
             Fibrous (fibroblastic)
             Transitional (mixed)
             Psammomatous
             Angiomatous
             Microcystic
             Secretory
             Clear cell
             Chordoid
             Lymphoplasmacyte-rich
             Metaplastic
2) Atypical meningioma
3) Papillary meningioma
4) Anaplastic (malignant) meningioma

b. *Non-meningothelial Cell Tumors*

Benign Tumors
1) Osteocartilaginous tumors
2) Lipoma
3) Fibrous histiocytoma
4) Others

Malignant Tumors
1) Hemangiopericytoma
2) Chondrosarcoma
   Variant: Mesenchymal chondrosarcoma
3) Rhabdomyosarcoma
4) Meningeal sarcomatosis
5) Others

c. *Primary Melanocytic Lesions*
1) Diffuse melanosis
2) Melanocytoma
3) Malignant melanoma
   Variant: Meningeal melanomatosis

a. *Tumors of Uncertain Origin*
1) Hemangioblastoma (capillary hemangioblastoma)

4 Lymphomas and Hematopoietic tumors
1) Malignant lymphomas
2) Plasmacytoma
3) Granulocytic sarcoma
4) Others

5 Germ Cell Tumors
1) Germinoma
2) Embryonal carcinoma
3) Yolk sac tumor (Endodermal sinus tumor)
4) Choriocarcinoma
5) Teratoma
     Immature
     Mature
     Teratoma with malignant
          transformation
6) Mixed germ cell tumors

6 Cysts and Tumor-like Lesions
1) Rathke cleft cyst
2) Epidermoid cyst
3) Dermoid cyst
4) Colloid cyst of the third ventricle
5) Enterogenous cyst
6) Neuroglial cyst
7) Granular cell tumor (Choristoma, Pituicytoma)
8) Hypothalamic neuronal hamartoma
9) Nasal glial heterotopia
10) Plasma cell granuloma

7 Tumors of the Sellar Region
1) Pituitary adenoma
2) Pituitary carcinoma
3) Craniopharyngioma
     Variants: Adamantinomatous
          Papillary

8 Local Extensions from Regional Tumors
1) Paraganglioma (Chemodectoma)
2) Chordoma
3) Chondroma
4) Chondrosarcoma
5) Carcinoma

9 Metastatic Tumors

10 Unclassified Tumors

* Kleihues, P, Burger, P, Scheithauer, B. *The New WHO Classification of Brain Tumours*, Brain Pathology 3: 255-268 (1993)

Drug and Treatment Abbreviations

The abbreviations listed below can help you translate medical reports, journal articles and research studies. Included are FDA-approved substances in current use, investigational substances which are offered only in clinical trials, and substances that are no longer available but which you will find referred to in medical literature.

This list is updated frequently. Call us at (800) 886-2282 for the most current version, or you can access it online at our Web site—http://www.abta.org.

Information about these substances can be obtained from your physician, through a PDQ search, a Medline search, or in medical textbooks.

Abbreviation	Substance Abbreviation or Generic Name
4-HC	4-hydroperoxycyclophosphamide
6MP	6-mercaptopurine
6-TG	6-thioguanine
ARA-C	cytosine arabinoside
AZQ	diaziquone
BCNU	carmustine
BG	0^-benzylguanine
BLEO	bleomycin
BPA	p-boronophenylalanine
	crisnatol mesylate
	cystemustine
CACP	cisplatin
CAMPTO	camptothecin, aminocamptothecin
CCNU	lomustine
CDDP	cisplatinum, cisplatin
CHOP	cytoxan/adriamycin/vincristine/prednisone
COP	cyclophosphamide/procarbazine/vincristine
CPDD	cisplatin
CRA	cis-retinoic acid
CSF	colony stimulating factor
CTX or CYT	cytoxan
DBD	dibromodulcitol
DEX	dexamethasone
DFMO	alpha-difloromethylornithine
DHAP	dexamethasone/cytosine arabinoside/cisplatin
DOX	doxorubicin
DTIC	dacarbazine

Abbreviation	Substance Abbreviation or Generic Name
FU	fluorouracil
GM-CSF	granulocyte-macrophage colony stimulating factor
HU	hydroxyurea
ICE	ifosfamide/cisplatin/etoposide
IFb, IFNb	interferon beta
IL	interleukin
LAK cells	lymphokine activated killer cells
	melphalan
MAB, MoAb	monoclonal antibodies
MeCCNU	methyl CCNU
MGBG	methyl-bisguanylhydrazone
MISO	misonidazole
MOP	mechlorethamine/vincristine/procarbazine
MOPP	nitrogen mustard/PCV/procarbazine/prednisone
MTX	methotrexate
OPP	vincristine/prednisone/procarbazine
	phenylacetate, phenylacetic acid
	phenylbutyrate
PCB	procarbazine
PCV	procarbazine/CCNU /vincristine
PRED	prednisone
	retinoic acid, isotretinoin, Accutane™
RMP-7	RMP-7
RU486	mifepristone
STZ	streptozotocin
SU-101	platelet derived growth factor-4
SUR	suramin
	thalidomide
	tirapazamine
TAX	taxol, taxotere, paclitaxel
TEPA	IV thiotepa
TIL	tumor infiltrating lymphocytes
TMX	tamoxifen
TMZ	temozolomide
TNF	tumor necrosis factor
TOPO	topotecan
TRA	tretinoin
VCR	vincristine, Oncovin
VENP	VCR/cytoxan/procarbazine or 6-mercaptopurine
VM-26	teniposide
VP-16	etoposide

Karnofsky Performance Scale

Score	Definition
100	Normal, no complaints; no evidence of disease
90	Able to carry on normal activity, minor symptoms of disease
80	Normal activity with effort, some disease symptoms
70	Cares for self but unable to carry on normal activity
60	Requires occasional assistance but is able to care for most of needs
50	Requires considerable assistance and frequent care
40	Disabled, requires special care and assistance
30	Severely disabled, might be hospitalized, but death is not imminent
20	Very sick, hospitalization necessary, active treatment necessary to maintain life
10	Dying

Glossary

accessible . . . . Tumors that can be approached by a surgical procedure; tumors that are not deep in the brain or beneath vital structures. Inaccessible tumors cannot be approached by standard surgical techniques.

acuity . . . . Clarity or distinctness of hearing or sight.

adenoma . . . . A usually benign tumor arising from a gland, such as a pituitary adenoma.

adjuvant therapy . . . . "In addition to." Therapy given at the same time or immediately following another
adjuvant treatment   treatment. The treatments work together to make each more effective.

age range . . . . In clinical trials, refers to the ages of patients who are eligible for a particular treatment. **Generally**, ages newborn to 24 months are defined as "infants," ages 24 months to 18 years are "children," ages 18 years and older are "adults."

agnosia . . . . Loss of ability to recognize objects, people, sounds, shapes, or smells. Usually classified according to the sense(s) affected (hearing, sight, smell, taste, touch). Symptom common to tumors of the parietal lobe of the cerebral hemispheres.

agraphia . . . . Loss of ability to write (a form of aphasia). Symptom common to tumors of the parietal lobe of the dominant cerebral hemisphere.

alopecia . . . . Loss of hair, baldness in areas where hair is usually present. A common side-effect of radiation therapy to the brain and some chemical therapies.

analgesic . . . . A medicine that reduces pain.

anaplasia . . . . Characteristics of a cell (structure and orientation) that make it identifiable as a cancer cell. Cells that have returned to a more primitive or undifferentiated form. Malignant.

angiogenesis . . . . The growth of new blood vessels from surrounding tissue into growing tissue.

angiogenesis inhibitor . . A substance that blocks the formation of new blood vessels. One of the biologic response modifiers under active investigation as a new treatment for brain tumors.

angiogram . . . . A diagnostic procedure done in the x-ray department to visualize blood vessels following introduction of a contrast material into an artery.

anorexia . . . . Loss of appetite.

anosmia . . . . Absence of the sense of smell. Symptom common to tumors of the frontal lobe of the cerebral hemispheres.

anterior . . . . Front or forward position.

antibody . . . . A protein produced by lymphocytes (white blood cells) in response to an encounter with an antigen. Part of the immune system.

antiemetic . . . . A medication that helps control vomiting.

antigen . . . . A substance, foreign to the body, which provokes an immune response: the production of antibodies.

aphasia . . . . Loss of ability to speak or write; loss of ability to understand speech or written words.

articulation . . . . Speech.

artifact . . . . Something artificial, a distortion that does not reflect normal anatomy or pathology, not usually found in the body. For example, in radiology, the appearance on an x-ray of a surgical metal clip that obscures the clear view of an anatomical structure.

ataxic gait, ataxia . . . . . . A clumsy, uncoordinated walk.

atonic . . . . Having no muscle tone, limp.

autologous . . . . Coming from the same individual, as opposed to being donated by another individual.

axial . . . . Position as it relates to the central nervous system (CNS). Intra-axial is within the CNS; extra-axial is outside the CNS.

benign . . . . Not malignant, not cancerous.

bilateral . . . . Occurring on both sides of the body; bilateral hearing loss is hearing loss in both the left and right ear.

biologic response . . . . . . A substance used in adjuvant therapy that takes advantage of the body's own natural
  modifier (BRM)   defense mechanisms to inhibit the growth of a tumor.

biologic therapy . . . . Treatment using biologic response modifiers (BRMs).

biopsy . . . . Examination of a small amount of tissue taken from the patient's body to make a diagnosis.

blastoma . . . . A tumor whose cells have embryonic characteristics, such as a medulloblastoma or a glioblastoma multiforme.

blood brain barrier . . . . . A barrier formed by blood vessels and glia which prevents some substances from entering the brain.

bone marrow . . . . The hollow center of bones where white and red blood cells and platelets are manufactured.

calcification . . . . Deposit of calcium. Associated with some types of brain tumors, as meningiomas, oligodendrogliomas and astrocytomas.

cancer . . . . Malignant tissue. It can invade and destroy healthy cells, and it tends to spread to distant locations.

carcinoma . . . . A malignant tumor that arises from skin or the lining of body organs, e.g. breast, lung, bowel. Carcinomas often invade adjacent tissue and spread to distant organs, including the brain.

catheter . . . . A thin, flexible tube. Can be part of a shunt. Used in the ventricles, other body cavities or vessels for the removal or insertion of fluids.

cell . . . . The basic living unit of body tissue. It contains a nucleus surrounded by cytoplasm and is enclosed by a membrane.

cell cycle . . . . The reproductive stages of a cell leading to cell division.

cell kinetics . . . . The amount of time it takes for a tumor to attain a determined size.

central nervous system . . Pertaining to the brain, cranial nerves and spinal cord. Abbreviated "CNS."

cerebellopontine angle . . The angle between the cerebellum and the pons, a common site for the growth of acoustic neuromas (vestibular schwannomas).

cerebral . . . . Refers to the cerebrum or cerebral hemispheres.

cerebrospinal fluid . . . . . The clear fluid made in the ventricular cavities of the brain that bathes the brain and spinal cord. It circulates through the ventricles and the subarachnoid space.

cerebrum . . . . The largest area of the brain, the cerebrum occupies the uppermost part of the skull. It consists of two halves called hemispheres. Each half of the cerebrum is further divided into four lobes: frontal, temporal, parietal and occipital.

chemotherapy . . . . The use of chemicals to treat brain tumors.

circumscribed . . . . Having a border, localized. Commonly describes benign tumors of the brain, such as meningiomas, pituitary adenomas and acoustic neuromas.

clinical . . . . That which can be observed in patients. Research treatments tested on patients, as opposed to laboratory or animal testing.

clinical cooperative . . . . A group of medical institutions cooperating to investigate new treatments.
    group

clinical trial . . . . An organized process for testing new treatments on patients using a pre-defined treatment plan. Clinical trials might be sponsored by the National Cancer Institute, the National Institutes of Health, pharmaceutical companies, or individual treatment centers.

CNS . . . . *See Central Nervous System.*

concave . . . . Having a hollowed surface, like the following: ⌣

congenital . . . . Existing before or at birth.

contralateral . . . . Affecting the opposite side.

control group . . . . Patients receiving standard treatment. In clinical trials, the control group is compared to the group that received an investigational treatment.

convex . . . . Having a rounded surface, like the following: ⌢

coronal . . . . Circular. In scans, an image from the top of a thin layer of the brain showing both the right and left sides.

cranial cavity . . . . The skull.

craniectomy . . . . Surgery performed on the skull where pieces of bone are removed to gain access to the brain, and the bone pieces are not replaced at the time of surgery.

craniotomy . . . . Surgery performed on the skull where a portion of bone is removed to gain access to the brain, and the bone is put back in place at the end of the operation.

CSF . . . . *See cerebrospinal fluid.*

CT or CAT scan . . . . **Computerized Axial Tomography.** An x-ray device linked to a computer that produces an image of a predetermined cross-section of the brain. A special dye material might be injected into the patient's vein prior to the scan to help make any abnormal tissue more evident.

cyst . . . . A fluid-filled mass. Usually enclosed by a membrane.

cytotoxic . . . . Capable of killing cells.

debulk . . . . A surgical procedure to decrease mass effect by removing a portion of a tumor or dead tissue. *See mass effect.*

decompressive . . . . Refers to a surgical procedure during which bone, tissue, or tumor is removed to lessen intracranial pressure.

dedifferentiate . . . . A mature cell returning to a less mature state.

density . . . . The amount of darkness or light in an area of a scan reflects the compactness of the tissue. Differences in tissue density are the basis for CT and MR scans.

diabetes insipidus . . . . . . A problem with water balance in the body causing excess urine production and great thirst, due to pituitary-hypothalamic damage.

differentiate . . . . The process cells undergo as they mature into normal cells. Differentiated cells have distinctive characteristics, perform specific functions, and are unlikely to reproduce.

diffuse . . . . Lacking a distinct border, spread out, not localized.

diplopia . . . . Double vision.

double blind . . . . A clinical trial where neither doctor nor patient knows which drug is being given.

drug delivery . . . . The method and route used to provide medication, for example, PO (by mouth), IV (intravenous), IM (intramuscular), intrathecal, intratumoral, spinal.

dura mater . . . . The outermost, toughest, and most fibrous of the three membranes (meninges) that cover the brain and spinal cord.

dysarthria . . . . Impairment of speech (articulation), caused by damage or disorder of the tongue or speech muscles. A symptom that can indicate pressure on the brain stem (medulla oblongata) or elsewhere in the posterior fossa.

dysphagia . . . . Difficulty in swallowing or inability to swallow. This symptom usually indicates tumors involving the lower brain stem.

dysphasia . . . . Language disorder. Inability to speak words which one has in mind or to think of correct words, or inability to understand spoken or written words. Symptom common to tumors of the dominant cerebral hemisphere, particularly the frontal, temporal, and parietal lobes.

dysplasia . . . . Abnormal development of cells or tissue, can be a precursor of cancer.

edema . . . . Swelling due to an excess of water.

efficacy . . . . Able to achieve the desired results, produces beneficial effects.

embryonic . . . . Undeveloped, related to the embryo.

emesis . . . . Vomiting.

encapsulated . . . . Localized. Refers to a tumor that is wholly confined to a specific area, surrounded by a capsule.

endocrine dysfunction . . With brain tumors, often refers to the decrease or absence of hormone production by the pituitary gland (hypopituitarism). In children, this can cause delayed sexual development and growth failure. Other symptoms of endocrine dysfunction include early puberty, anorexia and obesity.

epidemiology . . . . The study of the distribution of disease and its impact upon a population, using such measures as incidence, prevalence, or mortality.

etiology . . . . The study of the cause of a disease.

evoked potentials . . . . . . The use of electrodes to measure the electrical activity of nerves. Can be used as a guide during surgical removal of tumors growing around important nerves.

extracerebral . . . . Located outside the cerebral hemispheres.

extradural . . . . External (outside) to the dura mater.

extramedullary . . . . In reference to a tumor in the spine, between the meninges and the surface of the spinal cord.

familial . . . . Tending to occur repeatedly in family members, but is not genetic (inherited). Might indicate a susceptibility, or a common environmental influence.

fatigue . . . . Tired, weary, drained. Decreased ability to respond.

focal . . . . Limited to one specific area.

foramen . . . . An opening through a bone or membrane; the foramen magnum (literally, the large opening) is the hole in the occipital bone through which the spinal cord enters the skull and continues as the medulla oblongata.

friable . . . . Brittle, crumbles easily. A tumor that is difficult to remove in one piece.

gait . . . . Pattern of walking.

ganglia . . . . A mass of nerve tissue (gray matter), or a group of nerve cell bodies. Also refers to specific groups within the brain or spinal cord (as basal ganglia). Ganglion is the singular of ganglia.

gene therapy . . . . Treatment that seeks to replace or repair defective or abnormal genes. A biologic response modifier.

generic . . . . A drug not protected by a trademark. Also, the scientific name as opposed to the proprietary, brand name.

genesis . . . . The beginning of a process.

genetic . . . . Transferred via genes from parent to child, inherited.

GFAP . . . . **G**lial **F**ibrillary **A**cidic **P**rotein. This protein, found in microfilaments of glial cells, helps distinguish glial from non-glial tumors. A laboratory stain is used to test for its presence.

gland . . . . An organ of the body that produces materials (hormones) released into the bloodstream, such as the pituitary or pineal gland. Hormones have a widespread effect on the body and can influence metabolism and other body functions.

glia, glial tissue . . . . Supportive tissue of the brain, includes astrocytes, oligodendrocytes, ependymal
glial cells, neuroglia   cells and microglia. Unlike neurons, glial cells do not conduct electrical impulses and they can reproduce. The largest percentage of brain tumors arise from glia.

glioma . . . . Any tumor arising from glial tissue.

glucocorticosteroids . . . . Medications used to decrease swelling around tumors. Commonly called "steroids."

gray matter . . . . Gray matter, the "thinking brain," appears gray because it is composed of numerous nerve cells and blood vessels. The outer layer of the cerebrum—the cerebral cortex, and areas deep within the brain—the basal ganglia, are made up of gray matter.

growth factor . . . . A naturally occurring protein chemical that stimulates cell division and proliferation. It is produced by normal cells during embryonic development, tissue growth, and wound healing. Tumors, however, produce large, inappropriate amounts of growth factor.

gyrus . . . . An interior folding of the surface of the cerebral cortex. The precentral gyrus is a fold of the frontal lobe and the postcentral gyrus is a fold of the parietal lobe.

hemianopsia . . . . Loss of one half of the field of vision (the area that can be seen by each eye when staring straight ahead).

hemiparesis . . . . Muscle weakness of one side of the body.

hemiplegia . . . . Complete paralysis of one side of the body.

hereditary . . . . Transferred via genes from parent to child, inherited. Also called genetic.

herniation . . . . Bulging of tissue through an opening in a membrane, muscle or bone.

heterogeneous . . . . Composed of varied cell types.

homogeneous . . . . Composed of identical cell types.

hormone . . . . A substance produced by a gland and released into the circulation that affects the functioning of distant organs in the body. The pituitary is sometimes called the "master gland" because of the wide variety of hormones it produces and secretes.

hydrocephalus . . . . Hydro = water, cephalo = head. Excess water in the brain due to blockage of cerebrospinal fluid flow, increased production, or decreased absorption.

hyperfractionation . . . . . An increased number of smaller dosage treatments of radiation therapy.

hyperthermia . . . . The use of heat to kill tumor cells.

hypophysis . . . . Pituitary gland.

hypotonic . . . . Decreased muscle tone; limp muscles.

ICP . . . . Intracranial Pressure, harmful when increased.

ictal . . . . Refers to a seizure.

IICP . . . . Increased Intracranial Pressure.

immune system . . . . The immune system is the body's natural defense mechanism. It is composed of several different types of white blood cells and the products of those cells. The immune system's purpose is to attack and destroy harmful substances or objects it identifies in the body.

immunotherapy . . . . Use of the body's immune system to fight tumors. *See biologic response modifier.*

infiltrating . . . . Refers to a tumor that penetrates the normal, surrounding tissue.

informed consent . . . . . . The process in which a patient learns about and understands the purpose of a clinical trial, and then agrees to participate (or not). This process includes a document defining how much a patient must know about the potential benefits and risks of therapy before being able to undergo it knowledgeably. Informed consent is required by federally regulated studies. A patient who signs an informed consent form and enters a trial is still free to leave the trial at any time, and can receive other available medical care. *Adapted from "What Are Clinical Trials All About?," National Cancer Institute.*

infratentorial . . . . Below the tentorium.

interstitial radiation . . . . The implantation of radioactive seeds directly into a tumor.

intra-arterial . . . . Injection into an artery (that supplies a tumor).

intracavitary . . . . Treatment delivered into the space created when the brain tumor was removed.

intracerebral . . . . Located within the cerebral hemispheres (cerebrum). *See extracerebral.*

intracranial . . . . Within the skull.

intradural . . . . Beneath the dura mater.

intramuscular . . . . Into a muscle.

intrathecal . . . . Injection into the subarachnoid space of the meninges. Usually done by lumbar puncture.

intratumoral . . . . Injection into a tumor (usually performed during surgery).

intravenous . . . . Injection into a vein.

intraventricular . . . . Injection into a ventricle.

invasive . . . . Refers to a tumor that invades healthy tissues. Also called diffuse or infiltrating.

investigational new drug (IND) . . . . A drug that has been approved by the FDA (Food and Drug Administration) for investigational use only.

ipsilateral . . . . Affecting the same side.

irradiation . . . . Treatment by ionizing radiation, such as x-rays, or radioactive sources such as radioactive iodine seeds. Another name for radiation therapy.

labeling index . . . . The speed at which cells reproduce.

laser . . . . An acronym of **l**ight **a**mplification by **s**timulated **e**mission of **r**adiation. A surgical tool that creates intense heat and power when focused at close range, destroying cells by vaporizing them.

lateral . . . . On the side, as the lateral ventricles are located on both the right and left sides of the brain.

lethargy . . . . Sluggishness, drowsiness, indifference.

local . . . . In the area of the tumor; confined to one specific area.

lumbar puncture . . . . Spinal tap. Needle penetration into the subarachnoid space of the lumbar spine. Used to withdraw a sample of spinal fluid for examination. Also used to inject a dye into the spine prior to a myelogram.

malignant . . . . Cancerous or life-threatening, tending to become progressively worse.

mass effect . . . . Damage to the brain due to the bulk of a tumor, the blockage of fluid, and/or excess accumulation of fluid within the skull.

median survival . . . . Median means the middle value. An equal number of people live longer as die earlier than the median.

medulla . . . . The center or inner region. In the CNS, refers to the spinal cord and its continuation in the skull, the medulla oblongata.

membrane . . . . Thin layer of tissue covering a surface, lining a body cavity, or dividing a space or organ.

metastasize . . . . To spread to another part of the body, usually through the blood vessels, lymph channels, or spinal fluid.

metastatic brain tumor . . A brain tumor caused by cancer elsewhere in the body spreading to the brain.

mitosis . . . . Cell division, consisting of five successive phases, that results in two daughter cells.

mitotic index/activity . . . An indication of how fast a tumor is growing. The proportion of cells in a sample that are undergoing mitosis.

modality . . . . A method. Chemotherapy and surgery are two different treatment modalities.

monoclonal antibodies . . A biologic response modifier with unique "homing device" properties. Chemicals or
   (MAB)   radiation tagged to the MAB might be delivered directly to tumor cells. Or, the MAB itself might be capable of tumor cell destruction. MABs are mass-produced in the laboratory.

morbidity . . . . Complications directly resulting from a treatment.

motor . . . . Movement, control of muscles. The "motor cortex" is located in the precentral gyrus.

MRI scan . . . . **M**agnetic **R**esonance **I**maging. MRI is a scanning device that uses a magnetic field, radio waves, and a computer. Signals emitted by normal and diseased tissue during the scan are assembled into an image.

mutate . . . . Change in the genetic material (DNA) inside the cell.

necrosis . . . . Dead cells. A common feature of glioblastoma multiforme and other malignant tumors, including metastatic cancer to the brain. Caused either by lack of blood supply or irradiation.

neoplasm . . . . A tumor, either benign or malignant.

neuroectoderm . . . . The region of the embryo that eventually develops into the nervous system.

neuroepithelial . . . . The layer of tissue in the embryo from which the nervous system develops.

neuro-navigational . . . . . Pre-operative MRI information, fed into a specialized computer system, allows the
    system   surgeon to view 3-D images in the operating room during surgery.

neuron . . . . A nerve cell; it conducts electrical signals.

nervous system . . . . The entire integrated system of nerve tissue in the body: the brain, brain stem, spinal cord, nerves and ganglia.

nuclear atypia . . . . Some variance in appearance from a normal cell nucleus

nuclear medicine . . . . . . The branch of medicine that deals with the use of radioisotopes in therapy and diagnosis.

nucleus . . . . The center of the cell containing the genetic information (genes and chromosomes, DNA, etc). The appearance of the nucleus is used as a criterion to determine the malignant potential of a cell or tissue.

nystagmus . . . . Rapid, involuntary movement of the eyeballs.

Ommaya reservoir . . . . . A device with a fluid reservoir implanted under the scalp with a catheter to a ventricle. It allows for medication to be given directly to the CSF and into the brain.

oncogene . . . . A gene that, under certain conditions, can convert normal cells into cancer cells, e.g. the p53 and erbB genes.

oncogenesis . . . . The cause or production of tumors.

orphan disease . . . . A disease with an annual incidence, in the United States, of fewer than 200,000.

palliative care . . . . Caring for a patient by maintaining the best quality of remaining life. Also offering support and guidance to the patient and family.

palsy . . . . Complete paralysis.

papilledema . . . . Swelling of the optic nerve. Indicates increased intracranial pressure on the optic nerve. Also called choked disc.

paralysis . . . . Loss of muscle function due to injury or disease of the nervous system.

parasagittal . . . . Parallel to the sagittal (front to rear) plane.

parasellar . . . . Around or near the sellar region.

paresis . . . . Weakness.

paresthesia . . . . Abnormal sensations, such as tingling, burning or prickling.

PDQ . . . . **P**hysician **D**ata **Q**uery: a database that lists clinical trials sponsored by NIH.

permeable . . . . Allows substances to pass through. The blood brain barrier is selectively permeable, allowing only certain substances to enter from the blood vessels.

PET scan . . . . **P**ositron **E**mission **T**omography. A scanning device which uses low-dose radioactive sugar to measure brain activity. This is a limited-use diagnostic tool.

photodynamic . . . . A light sensitive drug is given through a vein and concentrates in the tumor. Then,
    radiation therapy   during a surgical procedure, a special light activates the drug. The activated drug
    (PRT)   kills tumor cells.

placebo . . . . An inactive substance. A harmless substance that has no biological effect.

PNET . . . . **Primitive Neuroectodermal Tumor.**

posterior . . . . The rear.

posterior fossa . . . . The posterior fossa is a shallow hollow of the occipital bone in which the cerebellum and fourth ventricle are located.

potentiate . . . . To make more effective.

primary brain tumor . . . . Original source of tumor is the brain rather than other areas of the body.

primary therapy . . . . The initial treatment.

primitive . . . . Undeveloped or in early stages of development, undifferentiated.

prognosis . . . . A forecast as to probable outcome.

proliferate . . . . To grow by cell reproduction.

prophylactic . . . . Preventative.

protocol . . . . An outline of care; a treatment plan.

proto-oncogenes . . . . . . Genes that are normally involved in cell growth and tissue repair, but are capable of becoming oncogenes.

proximal . . . . Located closest to the reference point.

quality of life . . . . Refers to the level of comfort, enjoyment, ability to pursue daily activities. Often used in discussions of treatment options.

radiation therapy . . . . . . The use of radiation energy to interfere with tumor growth, also called "irradiation."

radical . . . . Radical surgery is the resection of a tumor and a wide margin around the tumor in an attempt to remove any spreading cells.

radioresistant . . . . Resistant to radiation therapy.

radiosensitive . . . . Responsive to radiation therapy.

radiosurgery . . . . *See stereotactic radiosurgery.*

randomized . . . . Randomized clinical trials are those where each patient is selected by chance to receive one of the various treatment options.

recurrence . . . . The return of symptoms or the tumor itself, as opposed to a remission.

rehabilitation . . . . The return of function after illness or injury, often with the assistance of specialized medical professionals.

remission . . . . The disappearance of symptoms; the disappearance of the tumor.

resection . . . . Surgical removal of a tumor. Often used with an adjective, for example, macroscopic total resection—removal of all visible tumor; partial or subtotal resection—some visible tumor could not be removed.

residual tumor . . . . Remaining tumor.

respiration . . . . Breathing. To inhale and exhale.

risk/benefit ratio . . . . . . The relationship between possible risks and potential benefits of a treatment. Patients and their families must decide if the ratio is reasonable for them.

sagittal . . . . The front to rear plane of the body (chest to back).

sarcoma . . . . A tumor that arises from connective tissue, bone, cartilage or striated muscle. It spreads by extension into neighboring tissue or by way of the blood stream.

seizure . . . . Convulsions. Epilepsy. Due to temporary disruption in electrical activity of the brain.

selective . . . . Discriminating, choosy. A term used in relation to the blood brain barrier (which is selectively permeable), to vectors such as antibodies (where antibodies will bind only to particular cells, a trait that is crucial for effective drug or radiation delivery), and to other forms of treatment where uptake of targeted tissue only is important to successful therapy.

sella . . . . The saddle-shaped, hollowed extension of the sphenoid bone that contains the pituitary gland. The full name is "sella turcica."

sensitive . . . . Responsive, affected by.

sensory . . . . Sensation. The "sensory cortex" is located in the postcentral gyrus.

sequela (plural=sequelae) An affliction caused by a disease, a consequence of a disease.

shunt . . . . A drainage system. Spinal fluid flows via a surgically implanted tube from a ventricle in the brain into a body cavity. Used to relieve increased intracranial pressure caused by brain tumors that block the flow of spinal fluid.
  ‣ Ventriculo-atrial (VA) shunt: the tube empties into the right atrium of the heart.
  ‣ Ventriculo-peritoneal (VP) shunt: the tube empties into the abdominal cavity.

single blind . . . . In a clinical trial, the doctor but not the patient knows which drug is being given.

spasticity . . . . Increased involuntary muscle contraction (the opposite of hypotonicity).

spinal fluid . . . . *See cerebrospinal fluid.*

standard treatment . . . . . An effective, approved treatment—as opposed to an investigational treatment.

stereotactic . . . . Precise positioning in three dimensional space. Refers to surgery or radiation therapy directed by various scanning devices.

stereotactic radiosurgery A radiation therapy technique that uses a large number of narrow, precisely aimed, highly focused beams of ionizing radiation. The beams are aimed from many directions circling the head, and meet at a specific point.

steroids . . . . *See glucocorticosteroids.*

strabismus . . . . Imperfect eye coordination (crossed eyes) due to an eye muscle imbalance.

study arm . . . . One of the treatments offered in a clinical trial.

subcutaneous . . . . Beneath the skin.

superficial . . . . Close to the surface.

supratentorial . . . . Above the tentorium.

surgery . . . . *See resection.*

systemic . . . . Circulating throughout the body.

T1 weighted image . . . . . MRI image showing structures; CSF appears black.

T2 weighted image . . . . . MRI image showing water; edema and CSF appear white.

tentorium . . . . A flap of the meninges separating the cerebral hemispheres from the brain structures in the posterior fossa.

tinnitus . . . . Buzzing or ringing in the ear. Symptom common to tumors of the acoustic nerve.

tissue . . . . A group of similar cells united to perform a specific function.

tumor . . . . An abnormal growth. Tumors can be benign or malignant by cell type, or life-threatening (malignant) by their location.

tumor marker . . . . Substances found in blood or other fluids that identify the presence of a tumor, and/or the tumor type.

tumor suppressor gene . . A gene that stops the formation of tumors.

ultrasound . . . . Visualization of structures in the body by recording the reflections of sound waves directed into tissues. Can be used during surgery.

undifferentiated . . . . An immature, embryonic, or primitive cell. It has a nonspecific appearance, multiple nonspecific activities and functions poorly.

vascular . . . . Relating to blood vessels.

vascularity . . . . The blood supply of a tumor.

vector . . . . A carrier. A mechanism for delivering therapy to the cells of a tumor.

ventilation . . . . To supply air to the lungs.

vertigo . . . . Dizziness. Symptom common to tumors of the acoustic nerve.

white matter . . . . Brain tissue composed of myelin-coated nerve cell fibers. White matter carries information between the nerve cells in the brain and spinal cord. The inner portion of the cerebrum is composed of white matter.

Index

NOTE: *Italicized page numbers indicate illustrations.* **Boldfaced page numbers indicate the principal discussion(s) of the topic.**

oligodendrocyte, 10-11, *50*

oligodendroglioma, 37, **45, 50**, 52, 114

    oligodendroglioma, anaplastic, 50, 114

Ommaya Reservoir, 68, 71, 127

oncogenes, 21, 127

oncogenesis, 83, 127

optic canal, *53*

optic chiasm, *10, 11*, 11, 29, 34, 45, 51, *101*

optic glioma (*see* glioma, optic)

optic nerve (*see* cranial nerves)

orphan disease, 55, 127

P . . . .

papilledema, 25, 127. *See also individual tumors.*

parasagittal region, *48*

parasellar region (*see* sellar region)

PDQ , 78, 117, 127

Peacock System, 64

Pediatric Oncology Group, 103

perimetry, 34

PET scan, 32, **33**, 83, 127

photodynamic therapy, 60,127

pineal gland, pineal / pineal region tumors, 11, 28, **50, 51**, 66, *101*, **102-103**, 115. *See also* germ cell tumors.

    pineoblastoma, 51

    pineocytoma, 51

pituitary gland and tumors, *10, 11*, 11, 12, *14*, 27, *28*, **28**, 29, 34, *47, 51*, **51**, 61, 66, 67, 83, *101*, 116, 124

    pituitary adenoma, 51, 61, 116, 120

    pituitary carcinoma, 51, 116

pituitary-hypothalamic dysfunction, 83. *See also* endocrine.

pleomorphic xanthoastrocytoma, 37, 114

PNET, 42, 49, **51-52, 103**, 115, 128

polar spongioblastoma, 51, 115

pons, 9, *10*, 11, *14, 25, 26, 28*, 28, *44,* 44-45*, 47*. *See also* brain stem.

posterior fossa, 11-12, *12*, 26, 28, *48, 53*. *See also* infratentorium.

prevalence, 20

premotor area, *13*

primary auditory area, *13*

primary brain tumor, 15, 17, 18, 19, 21-23, 128. *See also individual tumors.*

primary motor area, *13*

primary somesthetic area, *13*

prognosis, **17**, 20, 128

prolactin, 11, 51

protocol, 75-79, 128

proton radiation (*see* cyclotron)

proto-oncogene, 21

pseudotumor cerebri, 52

Pseudotumor Cerebri Society, 52

R . . . .

radiosensitizers and protectors, 66

radiation therapy, **62-67**, 91, 128

radiosurgery, 64, 66-67. *See also* stereotaxy, stereotactic radiosurgery.

"real-time" imaging (*see* functional MRI)

recurrent tumor, 33, **52**, 62, 65, 66, 67, 71, 93

re-irradiation, 67

reservoirs, 58, 69, **71**

resection, 128. *See also* surgery.

reticular formation, 9, 12, 25

S . . . .

scans, *31*, **31-33**, 57, 103, 108, 113. *See also* CT, MRI, PET etc.

schwannoma (*see* acoustic neuroma)

second opinions, 56, **107**, 113

secondary brain tumor (*see* metastatic brain tumor)

SEER, 19, 20

seizures (convulsions), **24**, 26, 27, **95-99**, 104, 129

    absence (petit mal), 96

    atonic, 96, 121

    generalized, 96

    myoclonic, 96

    partial (focal), 41, 96

    tonic-clonic (grand mal), 96

sellar (sella turcica) region, suprasellar, parasellar, *11*, 12, 29, *48*, 116, 127, 129. *See also* hypothalamus, optic chiasm, pituitary, and individual tumors.

sex and sexuality, 82, 109, 113

shunts, **57-58**, *58*, 59, 129

ABTA Publications & Services Request Form

I. PATIENT EDUCATION PUBLICATIONS

Basic information
☐ A Brain Tumor—Sharing Hope
☐ Tumor del Cerebro—Compartiendo la Esperanza
☐ A Primer of Brain Tumors
☐ Dictionary for Brain Tumor Patients

Tumors
☐ About Ependymoma
☐ About Glioblastoma Multiforme and Anaplastic Astrocytoma
☐ About Medulloblastoma
☐ About Meningioma
☐ About Oligodendroglioma and Mixed Glioma
☐ About Pituitary Tumors
☐ About Secondary Tumors

For and about children
☐ Alex's Journey: The story of a child with
    a brain tumor (for children ages 9-13)
☐ When Your Child Returns to School

Treatments
☐ Gene Therapy
☐ Radiation Therapy of Brain Tumors: A Basic Guide
☐ Stereotactic Radiosurgery

Help and Resources
☐ A Bibliography of Books & Resources
☐ The Brain Tumor Survivor's Guide to the Internet
☐ Coping With a Brain Tumor
☐ Housing Assistance Resources
☐ Scholarships and Financial Aid Resources
☐ Transportation Assistance Resources
☐ Using a Medical Library
☐ Wish Fulfillment Organizations

Newsletter
☐ *Message Line*, 3 issues a year

2. SUPPORT GROUP INFORMATION
☐ Organizing a Support Group ("How-To" pamphlet)
☐ Listings of support groups by state (please tell us which state) _____

3. CONNECTIONS—A PEN PAL PROGRAM
☐ CONNECTIONS coupon (information we need to match you to a pen pal)

4. ABTA VOLUNTEER OPPORTUNITIES
☐ Send me information about volunteering for ABTA

Check the Publications and Services you would like and send this form to our office.

Name _____

Address _____

City/St/Zip _____

Phones & E-mail (optional) _____

American Brain Tumor Association
2720 River Road, Suite 146
Des Plaines, IL 60018-4110
Phone 847/ 827-9910 ▲ Fax 847/ 827-9918

This page left blank intentionally.

Emergency Alert

I have a brain tumor

My name is _____

Tumor type _____

I have had these treatments:

☐ Surgery   ☐ Chemotherapy

☐ Radiation   ☐ Biologic therapy

Date _____ *See reverse side* © ABTA, 1998

Emergency Alert

Emergency contact _____

Phone number _____

I am in a clinical trial   ☐ Yes   ☐ No

Contact this doctor _____

Phone number _____

See reverse side © ABTA, 1998

Emergency Alert

I have a brain tumor

My name is _____

Tumor type _____

I have had these treatments:

☐ Surgery   ☐ Chemotherapy

☐ Radiation   ☐ Biologic therapy

Date _____ *See reverse side* © ABTA, 1998

Emergency Alert

Emergency contact _____

Phone number _____

I am in a clinical trial   ☐ Yes   ☐ No

Contact this doctor _____

Phone number _____

See reverse side © ABTA, 1998

For each card, cut along dotted lines. Fold along solid line to fit in your wallet.

For additional cards, call our office at (800) 886-2282

This page left blank intentionally.